Praise fo ⎯

MW01102415

"As a vascular surgeon, I often see patients at their worst. Many of their health problems are the result of smoking and obesity. There is no doubt in my mind that the fountain of youth truly exists in the form of activity and healthy lifestyle. The results all point to less illness and longer lifespan.

*Hogevoll's down-to-earth **Muscle & Longevity** program outlined in **The Fitness Revolution** works for the 20-year-old on up to the octogenarian. I have personally brought his healthy approach of diet and exercise, with emphasis on weight training, into my own lifestyle. I recommend his methods to my friends and patients alike."*

Mark S. Peterson M.D.

*"The **Muscle & Longevity** program is an informed, rational program that is particularly helpful for middle aged adults who wish to embark on a healthier lifestyle. Hogevoll's program balances diet and exercise in a manner that facilitates the development of good habits while minimizing the chances of injury. Using his guidelines, I have established a pattern of healthy activities that I wish I had started earlier in life. Thank you Jerry."*

Larry F. Rich, M.D.
Director of Cornea Transplant Services, Casey Eye Institute, Oregon Health and Sciences University

*"In the 20 years I've been Jerry's physician I've watched his cholesterol plummet from 277 to 162. The **Muscle & Longevity** Program is a testament to what can be done with proper nutrition and exercise without the use of drugs."*

Michael W. Kelber, M.D. FAAFP

"Jerry Hogevoll and the folk featured in his fine book are living proof that old age does not have to mean geriatric. Some of these folk – who are also my friends – are as fit and vital now as when they were 30. You can be that way too by following Jerry's advice. It is never too late. Start today! We are still ahead of our time, Jerry, but the world is starting to listen."

Dr. Michael Colgan, PhD, CCN
President, Colagan Institure, Canada

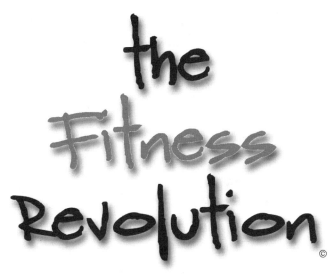

the Fitness Revolution©

The healthy way to get fit fast!

JERRY HOGEVOLL

Author, Fit Over 50

Copyright © 2002 by The Fitness Revolution Inc.

All Rights Reserved. No part of this book may be used or reproduced in any
manner whatsoever without written permission, except in the case of quotations
in articles or reviews. For information contact: Art Dept. 2517 S. River Road,Salem, Oregon 97302

Library of Congress Cataloging-in-Publication Data

Hogevoll, Jerry.
    The Fitness Revolution / Jerry Hogevoll
Includes bibliographical references and index.
ISBN 0-9672053-1-X

Printed in the United States of America

www.thefitnessrevolution.com • toll-free 877-581-8276

The Fitness Revolution

Contents

thing! One doctor advises us to eliminate carbohydrates and eat all the fat we want. Another tells us to eat right for our blood types. Another advises us to become vegetarians. Some prescribe weight loss, drugs, hypnosis, hormone replacement therapy or surgery. Others advise stimulants, aerobic exercise or electronic abdominal stimulators. Whom do we believe? What really works ?

Our government is doing little to fight the obesity epidemic. Don't expect this problem to get better soon. *Food processing is the largest manufacturing industry in the country and hence the most powerful.*

Over half of the head officials at the FDA (Food and Drug Administration) previously worked for the giant corporations that they

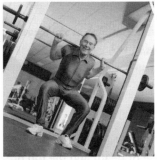

were hired to regulate. Most university research projects are financed by the food processing industry. Many politicians are financed by corporations that market processed and genetically altered food.

Food labeling is often fraudulent. Most of our drinking water is contaminated. Our soils are depleted of vital minerals. Over 80% of the food on supermarket shelves has been genetically altered. Many of our school food programs are

Jack Lalanne at age 86; his fitness philosophy was right all along.

controlled by fast food companies.

Having spent 25 years in the advertising business, I know the power of mass media. Most people believe what they read in the newspaper or watch on television. I made my living convincing people fast food is healthy.

The media is largely controlled by advertising dollars. Most new research findings are funded by the mega-corporations that market the product. It wasn't that many years ago that RJ Reynolds advertised that their *Camel* brand cigarettes reduced coughing and helped relieve sore throats!

At age 49, I made the decision to get in shape. I read every book, fitness article and fitness magazine I could get my hands on. What I found was a lot of confusing and contradictory information. I wasn't alone in my search for the "ultimate" fitness program. Americans spend 35 billion dollars each year on good marketing/bad science weight loss programs that don't work!

Those of us who are trying to get in shape are fed up with worthless exercise programs, misleading food labeling and bogus advertising claims. *The Fitness Revolution* has begun. Over the next decade, we'll begin to see more lawsuits and legislation against the corporate giants that are deceiving us, similar to the anti-tobacco movement of today.

I decided to ignore people who "talked the talk" and find people who "walked the walk". I have interviewed hundreds of the most fit middle aged people in the country. What I discovered is that although few of these elite athletes do everything the same, their fitness programs and diets share many key elements. *Their exercise routines and diets parallel the physical labor and diets of our paleolithic ancestors who lived 40,000 years ago!*

DNA studies have proven that the genetic make-up of modern humans is virtually identical to that of our caveman ancestors. That's why our bodies respond best to the same type of diet and exercise that our early ancestors had. We've inherited their genes, and we've actually changed very little.

My unique *Muscle & Longevity* fitness program combines these common diet and exercise elements into a proven synergistic six-part fitness program. I went from over 25% to 9% body fat in just 90 days on the program, and became a Natural Fitness Champion just three years later.

In the final analysis, we are all destined to meet our maker. I believe what's really important, when we reflect back on our lives, is that we gave and received love and that we helped others along the way. I'm blessed with the knowledge to be able to help those who want to help themselves. That's why I wrote *Fit Over 50* and *The Fitness Revolution*. I've heard a lot of people say they'd rather live well than live long. Personally, I prefer to do both! Making good choices regarding diet and exercise improves health and extends longevity. What is your health worth? *Ask the person who has lost it.*

chapter 2 # Are You Losing Muscle and Gaining Body Fat?

The human body is designed to live about 45 years. If it weren't for modern medicine and antibiotics, most of us baby boomers wouldn't be around if we had lived 10,000 years ago! Everyone knows our muscles weaken and we move slower as we age. Over time, our skeletal muscles develop many changes. The most noticeable is the loss of muscle mass. This is

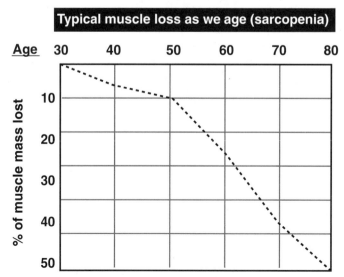

Typical muscle loss as we age (sarcopenia)

Age 30 40 50 60 70 80

% of muscle mass lost

10
20
30
40
50

because we lose muscle fibers and we never gain new ones, a condition called *sarcopenia*. Most of us start losing muscle fibers at about age 25. By age 50 our skeletal muscle mass is often reduced by 10%, and by age 80 approximately 50% of our muscle mass is gone. Because we are living longer, muscle loss is a serious problem.

Not only do we lose muscle mass, our muscles change. Humans have three types of muscles: fast fiber, slow fiber, and a hybrid combination of fast-slow fiber. In young people, these hybrid muscle fibers are scarce, less than 5%. In elderly people, our hybrid fast-slow fiber muscles average 33%. In young and middle aged people, skeletal muscles of fast and slow fibers are distributed in a chessboard fashion, whereas in the elderly, the fibers cluster in groups of either slow or fast cells. These recent findings have prompted many researchers to hypothesize the fiber types cluster in elderly muscle as a consequence of a complex process in which the muscle-controlling nerves originating from the spinal cord actually die. The nerve's muscle fibers are then left without any input, so they, too, atrophy and die unless they are reinnervated by another motor nerve.

If a muscle fiber is reinnervated by a nerve from a different motor unit type – for example, if a fast muscle fiber is reinnervated by a nerve from slow fibers – the muscle will transform to a slow fiber muscle. As we age, we lose more fast muscle fiber than slow muscle fiber. This means we gain a higher percentage of slow fibers as we age, and explains why a 12-year-old boy will outrun his grandfather in a short distance, but the healthy grandpa will defeat junior in a 10K.

Typically, men lose 6.5 pounds of muscle per decade after age 50 and women lose five pounds through menopause, then ten pounds per decade after that. Before individual fibers are lost to atrophy, they actually change in shape. In young people, muscle fibers are angular, whereas in the elderly, fibers are more rounded or even banana-shaped. A sedentary lifestyle plays an important part in sarcopenia. Have you ever heard the expression "Use it or lose it?"

chapter 3

How To Slow Sarcopenia

A s we age, our bodies slow the production of hormones necessary for growth. As we lose muscle, our metabolism (the rate at which our bodies burn calories) slows at the rate of about 10% per year after age 30. We gain body fat, become weaker, move slower and look and feel older. Around the corner lurk the threats of osteoporosis, falls and bone fractures.

Minimizing metabolic slowdown is essential for good health and longevity. Researchers at The University of Texas Medical Branch at Galveston have proven that losing muscle as a result of sarcopenia is not inevitable. Their three year study of 48 men found that muscle proteins are created and broken down at similar rates in both younger and older men. According to lead author Elena Volpi, M.D., Ph.D., now at the University of Southern California, "This is good news, because it means that any muscle mass lost with age is probably not due to some basic problem with the muscle cells."

Researchers concluded that vigorous exercise, dietary changes and supplements are essential to maintaining muscle, not treatments targeted at changing basic defects in muscle cell function.

Although many factors affect our metabolic rate, including genetics, gender and body composition, age will have a minimal effect on our metabolic rate if we control our body composition. *The only way to increase hormone production, stop this metabolic slowdown, and control our body composition is to build more lean muscle by lifting weights.*

Skeletal muscle is the most abundant tissue in the human body and also one of the most adaptable. Weight lifting can double or triple a muscle's size in 90 days, whereas disuse can shrink it by 20% in two weeks.

Many people associate weight lifting or bodybuilders with hormone enhanced, muscle-bound, professional freaks or portly power lifters from strongmen competitions. The definition of a bodybuilder, however, is any person who is trying to improve their physique and fitness level through weight training. Most bodybuilders follow natural, healthy diets, and incorporate aerobic cross training to build lean, muscular, healthy physiques and strong cardiovascular systems. The unique, synergistic *Muscle & Longevity* fat-to-muscle transition program is designed for men and women to achieve these same goals. It's never too late to start.

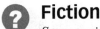 **Fiction**
Sarcopenia is a fact of life that we must accept as we age.

Fact
Weight lifting can prevent muscle loss and increase metabolism.

chapter 4 # How Weight Lifting Builds Muscle

Men have more and larger muscle fibers than women. This leads to the misconception that men "bulk up" more easily than women when lifting weights. On the contrary, male and female muscles hypertrophy (grow) at the same rate. To demonstrate this, a study was done on both men and women who, by using the same weight by proportion and performing the same routines, both achieved a 7% increase in arm circumference. The men only appeared to get bigger, because they had more muscle to begin with (men average 40% of their weight from muscle vs. 30% for women).

Don't worry about getting too muscular. This shouldn't be a concern unless you're blessed with incredible genetics or are muscular to begin with. If you do begin to bulk up, change your routine. A big advantage with weight lifting compared to other types of exercise is that you can target weaker body parts. Work strong body parts less and weak body parts more.

Contrary to popular belief, weight training does not significantly prevent loss of muscle fibers. *Scientific American* recently released new research proving that muscle fibers do not split to form completely new fibers. *Weight training does, however, increase muscle mass by thickening the individual fibers.*

Weight training exerts stress on muscles and tendons which starts a chain reaction to build more muscle. Genes stimulate the thyroid and pituitary glands to increase the body's release of natural growth hormones, including testosterone. This causes the muscle fibers to make more contractile proteins. More nuclei are required to produce and support the making of additional protein and to maintain a certain ratio of cell volume to nuclei.

Muscle fibers have multiple nuclei, but because nuclei within the muscle fiber cannot divide, new nuclei are donated by so-called satellite cells. These satellite cells proliferate in response to the stress of weight training, which causes "microtears" in muscle fibers.

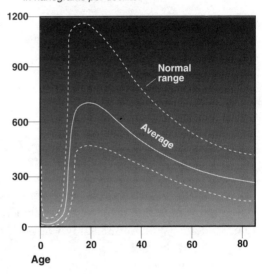

Testosterone Levels
in nanograms per deciliter

The damaged area attracts satellite cells that begin building proteins to fill the gap. As these satellite cells multiply, some remain as satellites on the fiber and others become incorporated into it. These nuclei become indistinguishable from the muscle cell's other nuclei. With the additional nuclei, the fiber is able to churn out more proteins and create more myofibrils, resulting in more muscle mass and a higher metabolic rate.

? Fiction

It is difficult for middle aged people to increase muscle and lose body fat.

! Fact

*Most middle aged people can dramatically alter their physiques in 90 days on the **Muscle & Longevity** Program.*

chapter 5 # How Weight Lifting Improves Our Sex Lives

S ome people are turned on by a fit body, but there are many more benefits weight lifting provides besides shapely legs, firm biceps, or a six pack. Nearly 80% of men over 50 years of age have experienced sexual dysfunction or decreased sex drive, and scientists estimate that 30-45 million women suffer from low sex drive. Notice the correlation between decreased sex drive and the percentage of people who are overfat?

Just a few years ago, doctors considered most cases of sexual dysfunction to be psychologically based. Today, due in part to better diagnostic tools and better understanding of sexual function, *nearly 80% of reported cases of impotence have physical factors as the primary cause of the dysfunction.*

The negative emotional state is more likely to be a reaction to the problem than the underlying cause. The leading cause of impotence is atherosclerosis (hardening of the arteries), *usually brought on by being overfat.*

We know that very low testosterone levels can impair sex drive and performance on men and women. We also know that increasing testosterone can enhance libido, and that weight lifting increases testosterone. This may explain why the majority of people on the *Muscle & Longevity* program report a remarkable increase in libido.

Not only do you reduce your risk of atherosclerosis, but getting fit also helps you to feel better about yourself. Mentally, you become sharper. Your body increases its output of testosterone, endorphins, adrenaline and growth hormones. As you become mentally and physically stronger, your stamina and *blood circulation improves everywhere*.

Maybe a better chapter heading would be *"Does sex improve our longevity?"* Scottish researchers at the Royal Edinburgh Hospital reported that sex is the key to looking younger. Their research showed frequent sex – at least three times a week – was second only to physical activity as a factor in looking younger than your age. Only monogamous sex helps, however, as infidelity and casual sex raise stress levels, thereby accelerating the aging process.

A ten year study at the University of Bristol, in the UK, found that men who had orgasms 3-4 times a week cut their risk of heart attack by 50%. Even men who admitted they barely move when making love received the benefits. The study also showed that sex is an excellent type of exercise for those recovering from a heart attack.

Another study showed 30 minutes of medium intensity sex burns 200-400 calories. So, if you don't like running, swimming, cycling or other aerobic activities, you might consider sex!

? **Fiction**
Most cases of sexual dysfunction are psychologically based.

! **Fact**
Nearly 80% of impotence have physical factors as the primary cause.

chapter 6 # Weight Lifting vs. Aerobic Exercise

F or twenty years we have been spoon-fed the notion that aerobic exercise such as running, biking or swimming is essential for achieving fitness. This simply isn't the case, especially after middle age.

Aerobic exercise: Prolonged, moderate intensity exercise that requires less oxygen than our cardio-respiratory system can replenish to the working muscles.

Our bodies burn fat for energy. Aerobic exercise makes our muscles work hard enough to require more oxygen, thus speeding up our heart rate. If you're working too hard and your muscles aren't getting enough oxygen, then you're working *anaerobically*.

It takes 10-12 hours of aerobic exercise to burn one pound of body fat. Fast twitch, or type 2 muscle fibers (the kind we lose with age), are most prone to hypertrophy, or growth. Slow twitch muscle fibers are endurance muscle fibers, less prone to growth when stimulated by weight training. Aerobic work alone affects primarily the slow-twitch, or so-called "endurance" muscle fibers.

Early man followed a pattern of hard physical acrobic and anaerobic work – hunting, lifting and carrying – for 2-3 days, followed by rest. Some have even likened such a schedule to modern weight training programs characterized by alternating sequencing of heavier and lighter lifting schedules.

Total fitness is composed of numerous components, including cardiovascular, skeletal muscle strength, flexibility, aerobic and anaerobic endurance, lean body mass, mental strength and self-image. Aerobic activity, generally speaking, does little for increasing the strength of the body's overall skeletal muscles.

Conversely, by using the same body parts over and over, aerobic work can actually create imbalances in the skeletal-muscle system, increasing the possibility of injury. Plus, aerobic exercises do little to improve flexibility, anaerobic endurance or lean mass.

Aerobic exercise is good for our cardiovascular systems, but it doesn't build enough muscle to prevent sarcopenia. Excess aerobics promotes decreased muscle protein synthesis, meaning aerobic exercise has a tendency to burn muscle, not fat, if done too much.

I used to do aerobic exercise for an hour, six days a week. After age 40, my body fat percentage crept higher each year. When I switched to a weight training program with aerobic cross training, my body fat dropped rapidly.

Weight training raises metabolism by increasing the percentage of lean muscle mass. Weight training also elevates metabolism for up to 24 hours, whereas aerobic exercise elevates metabolism for about one hour. Although some aerobics are necessary for a healthy cardiovascular system, _weight training, not aerobics, is essential for a fat-to-muscle transition._

Weight training not only makes the entire body stronger and more muscular, it provides better overall body symmetry. Let's use distance running as an example. Distance runners develop lean, muscular legs but usually have underdeveloped upper bodies, chests, shoulders, and backs. They often have poor body symmetry. Weight training isolates each muscle group, providing better overall bone-mineral density. Weight training enables us to improve any weak body part.

The _Muscle & Longevity_ high repetition, low weight lifting routines, known as circuit training, are aerobic. This routine strengthens our entire cardiovascular system and builds muscle at the same time.

Even though weight lifting is the key to preventing sarcopenia, aerobic exercise is an important element of the _Muscle & Longevity_ six part program. We can go from a fat-to-muscle transition without it, but it's not healthy. Aerobic exercise strengthens our entire cardiovascular system, increases oxygen delivery to muscles, helps digestion and accelerates fat burning.

Health Benefits from Weight Lifting

- *Improves balance* – strong muscles help maintain balance.

- *Improves bone mineral density* – reduces the risk of osteoporosis.

- *Decreases cholesterol levels* – increases HDL "good" cholesterol.

- *Increases glucose metabolism* – reduces the risk of diabetes.

- *Decreases blood pressure* – baby boomers who lift weights typically show a 3-4 point drop in resting systolic blood pressure.

- *Decreases arthritic pain* – increases joint range of motion.

- *Decreases depression* – A Harvard study showed over 80% of depressed baby boomers no longer met the criteria for depression after only 12 weeks of weight training.

- *Increases gastrointestinal transit speed (GTS)* – A three month study showed strength training increased GTS 56%, reducing risk of colon cancer.

- *Avoids muscle loss* – increases muscle mass for improved metabolism.

- *Improved cardiovascular system* – Weight lifting is aerobic and strengthens heart, lungs and circulation.

- *Improves brain function* – reduces the risk of blood clots and improves sugar regulation.

- *Stronger joints and tendons* – Weight lifting strengthens joints and tendons to help prevent injuries.

- *Better self image* – Weight training improves self image, and goal-setting standards.

- *Improved immune system* – *As the body gets stronger, so does the immune system. Not only will our body fight off serious diseases like cancer, we'll get sick less from common health problems like the common cold. If we get sick, it will be for less time and intensity.*

- *Improved sex life* – *Physical appearance can enhance sexual attraction. Weight lifting increases testosterone and improves blood flow everywhere, providing more energy and vitality.*

Fiction
Aerobic exercises like running, biking and swimming are essential for staying fit.

Fact
Aerobic exercise does little to improve flexibility, anaerobic endurance or lean muscle mass. Aerobic exercise has a tendency to burn muscle, not fat, if done too much. Aerobic exercise increases your metabolism for a very short period of time compared to weight lifting.

chapter 7

The Consequences of Obesity

T here are over 78 million of us baby boomers, and 75% are overfat! Health problems related to obesity cause over 300,000 Americans to die each year. That is 75% of all deaths in the country.

Leading Causes of Death in America

Rank	Condition	Percentage of Recorded Deaths
1	Heart disease	33.2%
2	Cancer	23.7%
3	Cerebrovascular disease	6.6%
4	Pulmonary disease	4.2%
5	Accidents	4.1%
6	Pneumonia & influenza	3.6%
7	Diabetes mellitus	2.3%
8	Suicide	1.4%
9	HIV/AIDS	1.4%
10	Homicide	1.2%
11	Liver disease	1.2%
12	Kidney disease	1.0%
13	Septicemia	0.9%
14	Atherosclerosis	0.8%
	All other causes	14.5%

Source: Centers for Disease Control.

According to the Center for Disease Control, overfat people are "America's biggest health problem." Being overfat is linked to nearly all the major killers, even accidents and suicide. Overfat people coming out of surgery face an increased risk of post-operative infection, by up to 700%. Being overfat weakens the immune system.

Over 60 million Americans now have atherosclerosis, the most dangerous result of our modern processed food diet and lethargic lifestyle. This progressive build up of clogged arteries prevents oxygen-rich blood from reaching the heart, triggering heart attacks and strokes. Although this disease was rare a century ago, today atherosclerosis is the leading cause of death in the U.S. for both men and women, and the single biggest risk factor to avoid.

Fifty percent of men and 63% of women who die suddenly from heart disease have had no previous symptoms. Over 80% of the people who died of heart disease did so during their first attack. You can check your chances of suffering a heart attack or stroke by using the risk index chart at the end of this chapter.

You Can Be Fit, But Not Healthy

Even though obesity is a major cause of clogged arteries, just because you appear fit, don't assume you're healthy. A processed food diet high in sugar and fat, and low in vitamins, minerals, fiber and other nutrients can lead to atherosclerosis. It is not uncommon to see people who appear fit, athletic and robust drop dead unexpectedly from heart attacks. It's like running a high performance engine with low octane fuel. The engine is going to carbon up and wear out much faster than it should. Athletic people require even more nutrients than sedentary people do.

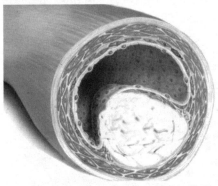

Atherosclerosis – deposits of cholesterol and other substances build up along vessel walls and become calcified, sealing off the passage of blood to the heart.

Early Detection Is The Key To Prevention

Most of us want to prevent heart disease, not wait for our doctor to tell us we need triple by-pass surgery. Modern science has made it fast and easy to show if you have – or are developing – heart disease, lung cancer, colon cancer, breast cancers or spinal problems. Coronary artery calcium scoring (CACS) is an advanced method available today to detect heart disease in its earliest stages.

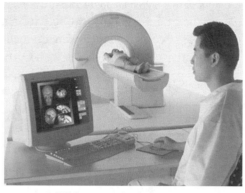

CACS uses non-invasive, high-speed computerized tomography to scan the heart and detect deposits along the walls of arteries. The test then produces a score that identifies your levels of

A CASC scan a is fast, painless and non-evasive method for detecting early heart disease.

deposits. Costs range from $500 for a heart scan to $1500 for a full body scan.

I have an athletic friend who exercises regularly and appears fit, but has had poor eating habits. He and his wife recently went in for a CACS and were shocked to learn he was developing heart disease (see their heart scans below). He has improved his diet and is now supplementing, which should stop and even reverse his condition.

CACS uses non-invasive, high-speed computerized tomography (CT) to scan the heart and detect calcium deposits along the walls of the arteries. The test then produces a calcium score that identifies your level of deposits.

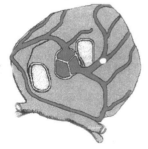

Healthy Heart
An axial view schematic provided by the CACS of her healthy heart.

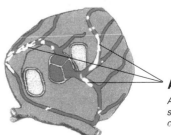

Atherosclerosis
An axial view schematic provided by the CACS of his heart showing calcification in the coronary arteries, an early indicator of heart disease.

People Who Exercise Live Longer

From 1982 to 1994, a study was done on 1,428 men investigating the effects of physical activity and mortality. They exercised only twice a week. The men were divided into 4 groups, depending on their activity level, Q1-2-3-4 with Q1 the least fit and Q4 the fittest. Over a 22 year period, from 1972 to 1994, 238 of the men had died. *There were about 150% less deaths in the Q3-4 groups compared to the Q1 group.* This study indicates you can significantly increase your life span by exercising a few times a week.

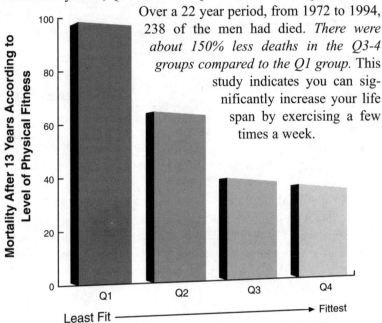

Type II Diabetes

The number of Americans with diabetes has reached 17 million, *a jump of more than a million in two years.* Type II diabetes accounts for an estimated 90-95% of those 17 million, and generally occurs during middle age. Type II diabetes is associated with obesity and inactivity, and impairs the body's ability to produce or efficiently use insulin.

Those who have high levels of blood sugar, but fall short of full-blown diabetes, are now considered to have "pre-diabetes", formerly known as "impaired glucose tolerance." According to Frank Vinicor, director of the diabetes program for the Centers for Disease Control and Prevention, "pre-diabetic patients who make lifestyle changes, exercise regularly, and lose 5-7% of their body weight can decrease their chance of developing diabetes by 58%."

How much body fat is dangerous? A 10% increase above ideal

weight can cause a 6-7% increase in blood pressure. This would be about 15 pounds on a 150 pound person.

Blood Cholesterol Types and Levels

Total Cholesterol	Less than 200 mg/dl	Good
	200-239 mg/dl	Borderline high
	240 mg/dl or greater	High
LDL Cholesterol ("Bad" Cholestrol)	Less than 130 mg/dl (less than 100 mg/dl if heart disease present)	Good
	130-159 mg/dl	Borderline high
	160 mg/dl or greater	High
HDL Cholesterol ("Good" Cholesterol)	Less than 35 mg/dl	High risk
	60 mg/dl or greater	Desirable

Cholesterol is an important indicator of cardiovascular disease. Just because you lower your "bad" cholesterol with drugs, don't assume you are out of the risk area. Your body fat percentage may be a better indicator of your risk.

Fiction

Smoking is the leading health problem in the U.S.

Fact

Obesity is now equal to smoking as the leading health problem, and is rising at an alarming rate.

Estimate your chance of suffering a heart attack or stroke

You can estimate your chance of suffering a heart attack or stroke by using this risk index. Remember, it's an estimate – not a diagnosis. Here's how it works:

Study each risk factor and its entire row. Find the most appropriate box for yourself and circle the point number in it. For example, if your age is 37, circle 3 points in that box. After checking out all 13 rows of risk factors, add the circled numbers. This total – your score – is an estimate of your risk.

AGE	10-20 years	21-30 years	31-40 years	41-50 years	51-60 years	61 and over
	1	2	3	4	6	8
HEREDITY (Parents' and siblings' cardiac health)	No family history of heart disease	One with heart disease after age 60	Two with heart disease after age 60	One with heart disease before age 60	Two with heart disease before age 60	Three with heart disease before age 60
	1	2	3	4	6	8
WEIGHT	More than 5 lbs. below standard	-5 to +5 of standard weight	5 to 20 lbs. overfat	21 to 35 lbs. overfat	36 to 50 lbs. overfat	51 to 65 lbs. overfat
	0	1	2	3	5	7
SMOKING	Non- smoker	Occasional cigar or pipe; live or work with someone who smokes	10 cigarettes or less per day	11-20 cigarettes per day	21-30 cigarettes per day	31 cigarettes or more per day
	0	1	2	4	6	10
EXCERCISE	Intensive job and recreational excertion	Moderate job and recreational excertion	Sedentary job and intensive recreation	Sedentary job and moderate recreation	Sedentary job and occasional recreation	Sedentary job; no special excercise
	0	1	2	4	6	8
CHOLESTROL LEVEL OR FAT % IN DIET	Cholestrol below 180 mg. Diet contains no animal or solid fat	Cholestrol 180-205 mg. Diet contains 10% animal or solid fat	Cholestrol 206-230 mg. Diet contains 20 % animal or solid fat	Cholestrol 231-255 mg. Diet contains 30% animal or solid fat	Cholestrol 256-280 mg. Diet contains 40% animal or solid fat	Cholestrol 281-300 mg. Diet contains 50% animal or solid fat
	1	2	3	4	5	7

GENDER	Female under age 40	Female 40 - 50	Female over50, male under 20	Male age 20 - 34	Male between 35 - 59	Male over 60
	1	2	4	5	6	7
SYSTOLIC BLOOD PRESSUE	Below 110	111 - 130	131 - 140	141 - 160	161 - 180	Above 180
	0	1	2	3	5	7
DIASTOLIC BLOOD PRESSUE	Below 80	80 - 85	86 - 90	91 - 95	96 - 100	Above 100
	0	1	2	4	7	9
STRESS	No mental-emotional stress	Occasional mild stress	Frequent mild stress	Frequent moderate stress	Frequent high stress	Constant high stress
	0	1	2	3	4	5
PRESENT HEART DISEASE SYMPTOMS	None	Occasional fast pulse and/or irregular rhythm	Frequent fast pulse and/or irregular rhythm	Dizziness on exertion	Occasional angina (chest pain)	Frequent angina (chest pain)
	0	2	4	6	8	10
PERSONAL HISTORY OF HEART DISEASE	Completely benign	Heart disease symptoms; not confirmed by physician	History of heart disease symptoms; examined by physician	Mild heart disease; no present treatment	Heart disease under treatment	Hospitalized for heart disease
	0	2	4	6	8	10
DIABETES	No symptoms; no family history of diabetes	Family history of diabetes	Impaired glucose tolerence	Dietary control	Oral medication control	Insulin control
	0	1	3	5	7	9

If your total score is:

6-14 = Risk well below average
15-19 = Risk below average
20-25 = Risk generally average
26-32 = Risk moderately high
33-40 = Risk dangerous
41-56 = Risk very dangerous
57 + = Risk extreme

If your score is above 25, work with your physician to reduce your risk factors.

PART

2

Our Diets Have Changed and We Haven't

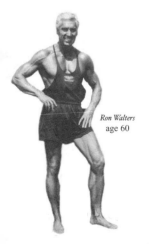

Ron Walters
age 60

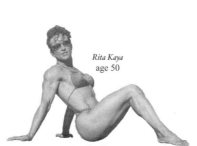

Rita Kaya
age 50

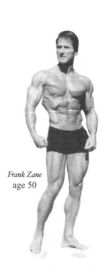

Frank Zane
age 50

chapter 8 # Blame Our Paleolithic Ancestors

T The obesity epidemic is a biological issue we can contribute to our Paleolithic ancestors (Paleolithic is a fancy name for the Stone Age or "hunter-gatherer" era). This era lasted from around 3.6 million years ago until the advent of farming known as the Agricultural era, around 11,000 years ago.

Understanding how our early ancestors ate during this period teaches us a lot about how our bodies have evolved, for our bodies haven't changed genetically in any meaningful way since we left this era. DNA research has proven human genetic composition is virtually identical to that of humans living 40,000 years ago. This is long before humans started farming. *That's why the human body still functions best on an eating plan similar to what our Stone Age ancestors ate!* There has been very little time, evolutionarily speaking, for our bodies to evolve to

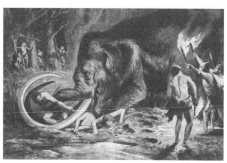

Man's genetic makeup has changed less than 1% in the last 10,000 years.

our new way of eating. Although 11,000 years may sound like an eternity, it's only 500 generations on the evolutionary clock since the Agricultural era began.

Granted, stone agers only lived to about 30 years of age, but they didn't die from today's modern diseases like cancer or cardiovascular diseases. They died from maladies like bacterial diseases that we now control with drugs and hygienic measures.

Americans eat over half their calories from new foods our ancestors didn't eat. Such foods include grains, dairy products, dried legumes, factory-farmed meat, processed foods, genetically modified foods, alcohol, separated fats (various oils), free salt and lots of sugar.

When an animal is fed food with which it has little evolutionary experience (hay to a bear for example), discordance occurs between these "new" foods and the animals' genetic profile. If the animal continues to eat this "new" food, the results are disease, dysfunction and early death. This same scenario applies to humans. *This mismatch between how we're programmed to eat and how we actually eat is the leading cause of obesity and disease in America.*

Americans prefer processed, high fat, sweet tasting food to satisfy our appetites. The problem is our bodies are too efficient at converting sugar to fat and storing fat. This is because only our early ancestors who had ample fat stores survived. Adequate fat stores were necessary to survive frequent famines and infectious diseases. Infectious diseases prevented nearly half of all infants from reaching their first birthday. Resistance to these diseases depended, in part, on how much body fat the child had. Just four degrees of fever raises energy needs to nearly 30% greater than normal. This is why individuals with a genetic propensity towards obesity, or who liked fatty foods, survived.

Even with these genetic characteristics to store body fat, our early ancestors were rarely overfat. They did a lot of hard physical work – lots of walking and running, moving things, digging and lifting. They worked hard to get a meal, or to keep from being a meal! Today, our bodies are still genetically programmed to protect us from famine. Our genes don't know there's a supermarket or a McDonalds just down the street!

The Hunter-Gatherer Era

Walter Bortz II, MD, is one of America's most respected experts on aging and effects of inactivity as it relates to the functioning of the human body. In his book *We Live Too Short and Die Too Long* he explains how our early ancestors first walked upright on two legs and left the jungles and moved to the plains. This was the beginning of the Hunter-Gatherer era. Bortz says "this was a historic event in the evolution of mankind. Food was close and plentiful in the jungle, but man had to work hard to get a meal on the plains. Only the strong survived.

Early man had to run down his prey and be strong to carry it back to camp. Early man had many disadvantages; he was small, slow, and had no killing jaws, teeth or claws like larger predators." So how did man survive? Man has the unique ability to run long distance. Big cats gave up the chase after a quarter mile or so, but early man kept game like antelope constantly on the run until they were totally exhausted and could easily be killed.

The Agricultural Revolution

The Agricultural Revolution, when we stopped following the food supply and started growing it, made life a lot easier. Our early ancestors didn't have to chase down an animal, kill it and carry the carcass back to camp anymore.

Smaller game, fruits and vegetables gradually began to replace larger game, which was now becoming more difficult to obtain. The shortage of large game animals is what researchers believe drove early man into farming, a move he made reluctantly. Wheat and grains slowly spread throughout the world, allowing man to get the calories and other nutrients he needed to survive the meat shortage and populate much of the planet.

The effects of this move from wild meat to grains as the foundation of the human diet had bad effects on our health. We lost an average of 6" in height, suffered a dramatic increase in tooth decay, bone malformations, infant mortality and acquired many new diseases unknown to previous Hunter-Gatherers including adult onset diabetes and coronary heart disease. *In general, our ancestors who ate grain were much less robust than our meat-eating ancestors that preceded them.*

The Industrial Revolution

Jethro Tull's invention of the seed drill in 1701 marked the beginning of the Industrial Age in America, because man no longer had to sow seeds by hand. With the advent of high-speed steel roller mills for milling cereals, nineteenth century America's diet problem became much worse. Modern advances in processing food for longer shelf life also contributed to the start of America's obesity epidemic.

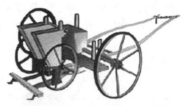

Jethro Tull's invention of the seed drill in 1701 marked the beginning of the Industrial age in America. Man no longer had to sow seeds by hand.

With the arrival of the Industrial Revolution, we didn't have to grow our own food any more (that was hard work too). We could just buy it at the local grocery store. As Bortz put it, "We became zoo animals." When zoo animals are confined and supplied with food they get fat and lose muscle tone – just like humans in the same scenario.

Our paleolithic ancestors lived on a well-balanced low glycemic carbohydrate, high protein, good fat diet. The carbs, proteins and fats were much different than what most of us eat today. They ate carbs in the form of beans, fruits, vegetables, roots and a few whole grain cereals. Most of the protein and fat came from lean wild meat.

? Fiction

Thanks to modern chemicals, herbicides and fertilizers, our modern diet is far superior to our early ancestors.

! Fact

Even though our modern crops are larger and sweeter, they lack the nutrients of the natural foods our ealy ancestors ate.

chapter 9 # Processed Foods

In Paleolithic times, virtually all of our carbohydrates came from fruits and vegetables known as paleocarbs. Today, Americans get less than one fourth of their carbohydrates from these foods. In the last few hundred years modern humans have invented ways to grind grains so fine that the bran is completely separated from the white flour. By the end of the nineteenth century, flour could be ground so fine that it resembled talcum powder, which is perfect for making soft, light, airy breads and pastries. Chemists and bakers know that the finest particle sized flour produces the best tasting and shelf-stable products.

Nutrients lost when refining whole wheat flour to white flour			
Protein	25%	Manganese:	82%
Fiber	95%	Selenium	52%
Iron, Fe:	84%	Thiamin (Vitamin B-1)	78%
Phosphorus, P:	69%	Riboflavin (Vitamin B-2)	81%
Potassium, K:	74%	Niacin (Vitamin B-3)	80%
Zinc:	76%	Pantothenic Acid (Vitamin B-5)	87%
Copper:	62%	Folate	59%

Our modern fast food diet comes from carbohydrates made from grain-based "over-processed" foods known as neocarbs. *Any natural food that has lost its nutritional benefits through processing is over-processed.* (Washing and cutting carrots can be considered processing.)

When we consume these over-processed sugars and starches, especially alone, without fats or protein, they enter the bloodstream in a rush, causing an immediate increase in blood sugar. The body's regulation mechanism shifts into high gear, flooding the bloodstream with insulin and other hormones to bring blood sugar levels down to

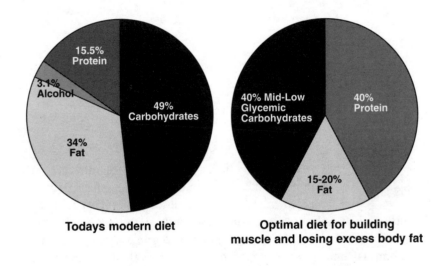

Todays modern diet

Optimal diet for building muscle and losing excess body fat

normal levels. A constant diet of neocarbs eventually disrupts this finely tuned mechanism, resulting in elements of constant over activity and eventually failure to respond at all. It's like crying "wolf" too often...eventually no one responds!

The situation is compounded by the fact that these neocarbs are also deficient in vitamins, minerals and enzymes, those bodybuilding elements that keep the glands and organs in good repair. When the endocrine system is constantly bombarded by neocarbs, numerous other pathological conditions soon manifest, such as: diabetes, heart disease, degenerative diseases, allergies, depression, behavioral problems and obesity.

The Pancreas Insulin Reaction

The pancreas is a vital organ that produces the hormone insulin. In simple terms, *insulin determines what we burn as fuel and store as fat.* When we eat high glycemic carbs the pancreas is "over stimulated" and produces too much insulin, resulting in high blood sugar (glucose) in the bloodstream. This blood sugar is stored as fat, because our body simply can't burn that much fuel that fast.

Ten years ago, fat was the biggest culprit for causing obesity in Americans. When Covert Bailey wrote his popular book, *Fit or Fat,* he said most Americans were overfat because they ate too much fat. He was right. Today, too much sugar and refined flour in our diet is the leading cause of obesity. This is because all the bad press about fat in the 80's prompted the food processing industry to reduce fat in processed food. Now they can label the food "fat free" or "low fat" and people buy it. *The problem is food processors have replaced fat with sugar or sugar substitutes.* They know most people like sweet food loaded with fat or sugar. It's the way Americans are used to eating.

Excess levels of insulin are thought to be the single most important factor in accelerating the aging process. High insulin levels affect our insulin resistance, blood pressure, body fat percentage, blood lipid levels, glucose tolerance, aerobic capacity, muscle mass and strength and immune function. When we lower our insulin levels, we improve all of these aging markers. We also reduce our hunger and food cravings, since our bodies can now tap into fat reserves for energy.

High glycemic processed foods are the worst foods we can eat when trying to lose body fat. A Glycemic Index of common foods can be found on page 45 or at www.diabetesnet.com/gi.html. With some exceptions, if food comes in a box or a wrapper, it's processed. Familiarize yourself with, and avoid, high glycemic processed foods.

Fiction
Too much fat in our diets is the leading cause of obesity in the U.S.

Fact
Because food processors are now replacing fat with sugar, sugar is the leading cause of obesity. The average American eats over 50 teaspoons of sugar each day, and the average teenager eats twice that much!

Glycemic Index

The glycemic index of foods is simply a ranking of foods based on their immediate effect on blood sugar levels from 0-100. It tells you if the food will raise blood sugar levels dramatically, moderately, or just a little.

Glycemic Index of Some Common Foods

INDEX GREATER THAN 100%			Garbanzo beans	61
(RAPID INDUCERS OF INSULIN)			Beets	64
Puffed rice	130		*50-59%*	
Rice cakes	135		Peas (frozen)	51
Puffed wheat	132		Potato chips	51*
Breakfast cereal	100+		Yams	51
100%			*40-49%*	
White bread	100		Navy beans	42
Whole-wheat bread	100		Peas (dried)	47
87-100%			Oatmeal (long cooking)	50
Carrots (cooked)	92		Sweet potato	50
Potato (russet)	98		*REDUCED INSULIN*	
81-90%			*SECRETION: 30-39%*	
Rolled oats (quick)	85-90		Black-eyed peas	31
Instant mashed			Milk (skim)	31
Potatoes	82		Milk (whole)	34*
Honey	87		Lima beans	35
White rice	82		*10-29%*	
Brown rice	82		Lentils	29
MODERATE INDUCERS			Soybeans	16*
OF INSULIN: 60-69%			Peanuts	12*
Raisins	65			
Spaghetti (white)	60		*high fat content	
Pinto beans	60			
Macaroni	64			

Fruit Juice

Most fruit juices are concentrated and contain high sugar content, whose glycemic index closely resembles fructose:

LOW	MODERATE	HIGH
Peaches	Pear	Banana
Plums	Orange	
Cherries	Apple	
Grapefruit	Grape	

PART

3

"Healthy" Food That's Killing Us

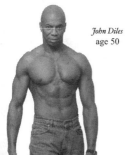

John Diles
age 50

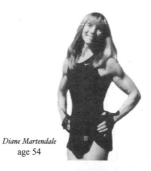

Diane Martendale
age 54

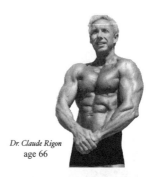

Dr. Claude Rigon
age 66

chapter 10 # Who Dictates The Food Pyramid, Anyway?

Many health conscious Americans are exercising, quitting smoking and following the government's food pyramid for dietary advice. Then why are more people than ever dying from an ever-increasing toll of new degenerative diseases? Something is terribly wrong.

Recently, the Department of Agriculture issued new nutritional guidelines in the form of a food pyramid. *The biggest problem is that the pyramid guidelines make no distinction between fats, proteins, and carbohydrates, maintaining that they have equal nutritional value regardless of how much or how little they are processed.* There is no reference showing whole grains or refined; between natural and genetically modified foods, between free range and factory-farmed livestock. Not a hint about health problems caused by factory-farmed dairy, eggs, or beef.

The food pyramid recommends a diet based on grains – breads, pasta, and cereals – along with fruits and vegetables. The guidelines recommend only small amounts of protein foods – meat, fowl, fish, nuts and legumes. The pyramid also suggests we should reduce sweets and fats.

This diet may keep us alive, but most people will not be healthy or fit on it and we certainly can't build muscle eating this way. For many people this diet contains several health risks. As I mentioned earlier, when humans first switched from a high protein to a grain diet about 11,000 years ago, the health effects were not good. Many people do poorly on grains, especially when trying to lose body fat.

The new RDA of calories from fat is 25%. Most humans who eat this much fat are going to be overfat! People of any age should eat no more than 20% of their daily calories from good fat and no more than 10-15% when trying to reduce body fat. (The food pyramid makes no distinction between good fat and processed fat).

The *Journal of the American Medical Association* reports one in every three Americans is obese by 40% or more. This is because the average American gets about 80% of their daily calories from "bad" fat and sugar. *This is three times the fat and sugar we should be eating.* Maybe all processed food should be required to contain a warning label, much like tobacco products. ***WARNING! This product may be hazardous to your health.***

Who sets the food pyramid anyway? The researchers, government officials, FDA, Department of Agriculture and other various government and quasi-government agencies. How could they have omitted so many important diet factors that negatively influence our health?

Over half the leading officials at the FDA have previously worked for the food processing industry. It makes one wonder how much influence the powerful food processing industry exerts on the politicians.

Many trained professionals struggle with the food pyramid and the RDA. In a 1995 study published in the *Journal of the American Dietetics Association*, dietitians were asked to design diets that met the 1989 RDAs and 1990 dietary guidelines, while providing 2200-2400 calories. Even using special software designed for creating a healthy diet, these trained dietitians were unable to accomplish the given objective!

The government is continuing to make steps in the right direction regarding the food pyramid, but it's time they eliminate "politically correct" nutritional guidelines.

chapter 11

Sugar and Sugar Substitutes

O ur early ancestors didn't eat refined sugars. They ate foods high in fiber and nutrients that contained limited natural sugars. Thanks to processed foods, the average American consumes over 150 pounds of added sugar each year, or *53 teaspoons of sugar every day*. The average teenage boy eats twice that much!

There are over 100 health hazards (including obesity) caused directly by sugar. Too much sugar overworks, exhausts and weakens the immune system, depleting essential hormones and causing an imbalance in body chemistry. Just two teaspoons of sugar can change blood chemistry and throw our bodies out of balance (homeostasis). This imbalance prevents white blood cells from fighting disease and opens the door to innumerable infectious and degenerative diseases. Sugar is added to most processed food we eat. Even foods like catsup, crackers, and non-dairy creamer contain sugar.

Food manufacturers use sugar in food that doesn't even need to be sweetened simply because sugar is a cheap filler. Even people who read nutritional labels looking for low fat foods often buy foods high in sugar or sugar substitutes without realizing it. Sugar is listed in grams, not teaspoons, on the nutritional label – and with approximately four grams in a teaspoon of sugar, this can add up quickly.

Popular soft drinks like Coca Cola, Odwalla lemonade, Ocean Spray CranApple, and even Ultra-Slim Fast juice drinks each contain over ten teaspoons of sugar! If you eat two cups of Frosted Flakes for breakfast you will have eaten ten teaspoons of sugar. Even a 6-ounce serving of fruit yogurt has seven teaspoons of sugar or honey. Most people are shocked when they calculate how much sugar they eat each day. Read food labels and learn to recognize and avoid sugar in its numerous forms. Look for words that end with "ose" including sucrose, dextrose, sucralose, galactose, maltose, glucose or fructose. Other sugar products include molasses, corn syrup, and fruit juice concentrate.

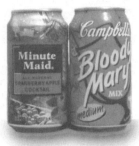

Many popular "fruit" juices and soft drinks contain over ten teaspoons of sugar.

More than 5,000 schools in the U.S. have contracts with fast food companies to provide food for their cafeterias and/or vending machines. It's no wonder our children and grandchildren are facing an ever-increasing obesity epidemic!

Artificial sweeteners

The artificial sweetener market is a 1.5 billion dollar per year industry. About 70-80% of that market is made up of soft drink sweeteners, of which aspartame (NutraSweet) has a near monopoly.

Americans consume 30 pounds of artificial sweeteners per person, per year. Non-caloric artificial sweeteners are not replacing, but rather supplementing, conventional sweeteners. As the consumption of sugar has risen, so has the consumption of artificial sweeteners. Artificial sweeteners were originally developed for weight loss but research has proven that they increase the appetite by stimulating the salivary glands, thus defeating their original purpose.

Popular sugar substitutes include saccharin (Sweet'n Low), aspartame (Equal, NutraSweet), Sucralose (Splenda) and Stevia. Studies have shown saccharin, aspartame and sucralose can cause many serious health problems, including cancer in laboratory animals.

Sucralose, marketed under the name Splenda, is the up-and-coming "next generation" of high intensity sugar substitutes. Sucralose is produced by chlorinating sugar, or chemically changing the structure of the sugar molecules. While limited testing has been done on Sucralose, the initial results are not good. The Sucralose Toxicity Information Center concludes that, "While it is unlikely that sucralose is as toxic as Monsanto's aspartame, it is clear from the hazards seen in pre-approval research and from its chemical structure that years or decades of use may contribute to serious chronic immunological or neurological disorders."

Healthy Sugar Substitute

Stevia, a small shrub in the chrysanthemum family and native to the highlands of South America, is a healthy sugar substitute. Stevia has a taste that is anywhere from 15 to 300 times sweeter than sugar, depending on the way it is processed. While many people like the taste of Stevia, some detect a licorice taste, or find it leaves a slightly bitter aftertaste. Many brands taste different because they use fillers like Erythritol, a natural filler from wheat or corn. I prefer pure stevia extract powder like KAL dietary supplement.

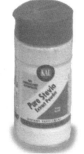

Although accepted for general use in Japan and Brazil as a natural sweetening agent, Stevia's use in the U.S. is limited to dietary supplements only. Although more long-term study is needed, I believe these laws are purely political to keep Stevia out of the lucrative U.S processed food market dominated by other artificial sweeteners.

Stevia is a healthy natural sugar substitute

Is honey or raw sugar better than refined sugar?

There is no health benefit to substituting raw sugar or honey for sugar. Both honey and raw sugar have a glycemic index of about 60, the same as refined sugar. If the honey is glucose enriched it has an even higher glycemic index rating. There are negligible quantities of other nutrients in honey. Honey is basically a mixture of glucose and fructose. These two simple sugars are bound together as a disaccharide (double sugar) in refined sugar. The end result of digestion in the small intestine is similar for both honey, raw sugar and refined sugar.

 Fiction
Soft drinks are a healthy alternative in place of water.

 Fact
Soft drinks contain lots of sugar and/or artificial sweeteners.

chapter 12

Red Meat: It's Not What It Used To Be

Most anthropologists agree that the average stone age diet consisted of 40-65% of total daily calories from protein (mostly red meat) but the source and nutrient content of their meat was much different than modern factory-farmed meat. Their meat was lean, wild game that averaged only 4% fat. *Most of today's factory-farmed domesticated beef averages 25-35% fat.*

The lowfat, wild red meat our ancestors ate meant fewer calories, similar to ocean fish or free range bison. Wild game contains more protein per serving than domestic meats. Wild game like our early ancestors ate – bison, horse, antelope, mammoth, mastodon and elk – is much healthier than factory-farmed livestock. Wild game contains two to three times more cholesterol-lowering polyunsaturated fats and almost five times more Omega-3 fatty acids than meat from grain-fed, factory-farmed domestic livestock.

Factory-farmed animals are given steroids, growth hormones and antibiotics to increase bottom line profits. Farmers don't get paid by the amount of nutrients the meat contains, they get paid by the pound. Growing animals faster, larger and fatter increases profits and supplies Americans with the high fat, sweet tasting meat we have grown accustomed to.

Most of the feed that factory-farmed livestock eat is genetically altered and contains high levels of pesticides and herbicides. This is because the grain, corn and soybeans used for the feed is sprayed routinely, even while growing, with special biotech herbicides. We assimilate these toxins when we eat the meat.

I eat a lot of free range bison, elk and venison. Bison is close to the wild red meat our early ancestors ate and can be readily purchased. Cooked bison looks and tastes like beef. Bison has more protein than beef and one-third the fat of skinless chicken. A four-ounce serving of bison filet mignon has only 1/2 gram of fat.

Bison is high in essential folic acid, which is necessary for the production of healthy red blood cells and for making new cells in the body, especially along your digestive tract. Bison is also higher in iron, thiamin and essential fatty acids.

I made more muscle gains in one year eating bison and venison than I did in the previous three years eating fish and occasional lean beef and I maintained low body fat. I ate five ounces of bison or wild meat three times a week. Bison is an excellent form of protein and can be substituted for fish or poultry, even when "cutting" body fat.

If you don't like bison or wild meat, eat natural, organic or range fed beef sparingly. Buy lean cuts from the loin and the round or ground meat that is at least 90% lean. Beware of deceptive labeling practices that say "free range" or "natural", as they usually aren't (See chapter 19, Labeling Fraud). For suppliers of free range bison see Suppliers Directory, page 195.

❓ Fiction
Red meat is high in fat.

❗ Fact
Most wild free range meat like bison, elk and venison have less fat than fish and 2-3 times more cholesterol-lowering polyunsaturated fats than factory-farmed livestock.

Factory-farmed beef vs. free range bison comparison

Beef filet mignon

4 oz   220 calories   21 gr. Protein   11.2 gr. Fat

Bison filet mignon

4 oz   110 calories   25 gr. Protein   .5 gr. Fat

Bison Nutritional Profile
3 1/2 oz. cooked lean Bison

	Fat (gm)	Calories (kcal)	Cholesterol (mg)
Bison	2.42	143	82
Beef	9.28	211	86
Pork	9.66	212	86
Chicken (skinless)	7.41	190	89
Lamb	9.64	200	87
Veal	6.94	176	106
Venison	3.20	158	112
Ostrich	3.00	140	83

USDA Handbook 8-5:8-10:8-13:8-17, nutritionalist TV

chapter 13 # Like It Or Not, Man Is An Omnivore

N ot a single hunter-gatherer society survived solely on plant foods. Only 14% of those early societies obtained more than 50% of their food from wild plants. Lean game and fish were the staple foods of the time.

In the 1950's and even now, researchers mistakenly link saturated fat from red meat to heart disease. The message many health professionals and doctors get is that meat causes cancer and heart disease. This notion is further ingrained by many diet gurus promoting vegan and vegetarian diets.

Scientists have now discovered that saturated fat from animal protein, as proven by the evolutionary diet, is quite healthful for humans. Red meat is rich in iron and zinc, both of which play

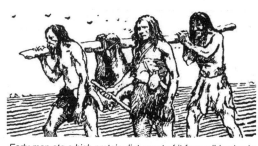

Early man ate a high protein diet, most of it from wild animals

important roles in the body's use of essential fatty acids. *Health problems are caused by the steroids, growth hormones, antibiotics and genetically altered feed used in raising factory-farmed livestock.*

The genetically altered grains fed to domesticated animals turn healthful lean protein with a proper balance of fatty acids into a nutritional nightmare that promotes coronary heart disease and various types of cancer.

Our primitive ancestors subsisted on a diet composed largely of meat and fat, augmented with vegetables, fruits, seeds and nuts. Recent research by noted anthropologists Dr. Emmanuel Cheraskin and Dr. Weston Price have shown early man, who subsisted on high protein diets, had excellent bone structure, heavy musculature and flawless teeth. Studies show that agricultural man, whose diet consisted mostly of grains and legumes, suffered from bone problems and diseases.

John Robbins, author of *The Food Revolution*, claims vegetarians live longer than meat eaters. This may be true in the U.S., but it's because most Americans eat factory-farmed livestock. Actually, the longest living ethnic groups eat diets high in animal products. These groups include the Russians from the Caucasus Mountains, the Soviet Georgian population and the Vilcabamba inhabitants of Ecuador. *On the other hand, many vegetarian ethnic groups like the inhabitants of southern India have the shortest life spans in the world.*

It is difficult to obtain adequate protein on a vegetarian diet and such a diet often leads to mineral deficiencies as well. The vegetarian diet lacks the fat-soluble catalysts needed for mineral absorption. In addition, the phytates in grains, unless properly soaked, block mineral absorption. Zinc, iron, calcium and other minerals are more easily absorbed from animal sources than grain sources. Usable vitamin B12 occurs only in animal products. Because grains and vegetables eaten alone cannot supply complete amino acids, vegetarians must balance the two at every meal.

Vegetarians tend to be deficient in phosphorus, as meat is the primary dietary source. This is one reason a vegetarian diet has been linked to tooth decay. *Research studies now prove wild or free-range red meat actually lowers blood cholesterol levels and reduces the risk for coronary heart disease.* Recent studies done at University of Western Ontario and Harvard School of Public Health show that "elevated protein (from lean meat) reduces the risk of stroke and hypertension and helps boost survival time for women with breast cancer. A high protein diet also improves or normalizes insulin metabolism in Type II diabetics."

Humans have a balanced PH, containing both acid and akaline tissues. If we were meant to be vegetarians, we wouldn't produce any acid. We'd be totally alkaline like herbivores (plant eating animals like cattle or horses). All foods that contain protein are digested in an acid base. Carbohydrate foods such as fruits, grains and vegetables are digested in an alkaline base. This acid/alkaline base is our genetic make up which makes us omnivores (creatures that eat everything).

Vegetarians often have difficulty maintaining a proper acid-alkaline balance in the blood and tissues because they lack essential vitamins and minerals necessary for this complex regulatory mechanism. Even minor deficiencies in these essential minerals can result in serious health problems.

If you could stick your hand down your throat into your stomach, your fingers would soon dissolve. That's because hydrochloric acid plays an important part in food digestion. This strong acid helps us digest protein foods as well as all others. *Another important benefit of this acid is that it kills potentially dangerous bacteria and viruses.* That's why dogs can drink toilet water without getting sick. If our acid levels are high enough, our bodies will destroy most pathogens.

As our modern society has switched towards more carbohydrates and less meat and protein in our diets, we have become more alkaline. As a result, the acid in our stomachs has become weaker resulting in increased illnesses from the pathogens in our food and water.

If we were herbivores, we would manufacture cellulace, an enzyme that an herbivore produces to digest plants. For example, a rabbit or horse will secrete cellulace to absorb cellulose. Humans don't manufacture cellulace, never did – never will.

It is especially important for older men to eat red meat to protect their testosterone levels. According to the Journal of *Clinical Endocrinology and Metabolism,* which conducted a study of 1,552 men, ages 40-70, "Diets low in protein lead to a reduction in the availability of testosterone, causing loss of muscle mass, red cell mass and bone density in men."

There are several reasons people become vegetarians or vegans. (Vegetarians don't eat meat, vegans don't eat any animal products.) Some abstain from animal products because of the carcinogens in factory-farmed livestock or the inhumane way the animals are raised and slaughtered. Some simply don't like the taste, or have trouble digesting protein. Some vegans believe they are attaining spiritual enlightenment.

I respect vegetarians and vegans for all of these reasons but the fact is animal products are essential for optimum health, growth, and healthy reproduction. Animal products contain complete proteins and plants don't. If we eat the same type of lean, free range or wild meat we're genetically programmed to eat, we'll get the nutrients we need, without the toxins.

If you're a vegetarian or vegan for whatever reason, it's going to be hard to get enough protein, minerals and vitamins in natural form. Your liver is going to have to work a lot harder to come up with the right combinations for your body to use. I suggest you get advice from a nutritionist and carefully monitor your daily diet. You'll have to stick with bee pollen, legumes, nuts, tofu, soy or whey protein supplements, amino acids and spirulina.

Spirulina is a microalgae 60% all-vegetable protein, rich in beta carotene, iron, vitamin B-12 and the rare essential fatty acid, GLA. It offers a striking profile of vitamins, minerals and phytonutrients.

❓ Fiction
We should all be vegetarians.

❗ Fact
Our early ancestors subsisted on a diet composed largely of meat. The problem is modern factory-farmed meat is very different than the free-range wild meat we're genetically programmed to eat. Man didn't start farming until 11,000 years ago and suffered many health problems switching from a high protein diet to a high carbohydrate diet.

chapter 14 **Whole Grains**

A nnual grain consumption has increased over 60 pounds per person in the last fifteen years. The RDA and many nutritionists may mean well when they suggest we consume whole grains but this is misleading. Although our early ancestors ate whole grains, they didn't consume them in the same form we do in modern times. Our ancestors soaked or fermented their grains before making them into porridge or breads. Today's modern grains include refined flours, polished rice, quick-rise breads, granolas and other over-processed fast food concoctions.

The practice of fermenting concurs with what modern science has discovered about grains. All grains contain phytic acid (an organic acid in which phosphorus is bound) in the outer layer or bran. Untreated phytic acid can combine with calcium, magnesium, copper, iron and especially zinc in the intestinal tract and block their absorption. This is why people who consume diets high in unfermented whole grains often have serious mineral deficiencies and bone loss.

Scientists know the proteins in grains, especially gluten, are difficult to digest. Animals that feed on grain have as many as four stomachs. Humans have only one stomach and a much shorter intestine compared to herbivorous animals. These features allow us to pass animal products before they putrefy in the gut but make us less well adapted to a diet high in grains. By letting the grains soak overnight in warm water, we let the friendly bacteria do some of our digesting for us, much like is done in the extra stomachs of the herbivores.

Soaking allows enzymes to break down and neutralize phytic acid. Soaking also neutralizes enzyme inhibitors present in all seeds and produces more beneficial enzymes. This enzyme action also increases the amounts of many vitamins. This simple practice of soaking cracked or rolled cereal grains overnight will vastly improve their nutritional benefits.

Bread

Modern bread makes the sandwich possible. Old style sourdough, slow-rise breads are too dense and hard for sandwich lovers. It was the advent of baker's yeast which produces a quick rise in a short time period so the phytates in whole grains are not properly neutralized that allowed bakers to produce the soft bread that Americans prefer. Unfortunately, both whole grain and refined flour breads are unhealthy, especially when dough conditioners and preservatives are added.

However, there are a few breads made with baker's yeast that have allowed the grains to sprout or sour. Although not recommended for a daily diet, these breads are much healthier. Look for sourdough or sprouted grain breads, made with a variety of grains, in the freezer compartment of your local health food store. Although pita bread isn't made with yeast, the dough isn't allowed to sour so it should be avoided.

Breakfast Cereals-Granola

Boxed breakfast cereals like Cheerios and Wheaties are made by an extrusion process, where little flakes or fancy shapes are formed at high temperatures and pressures. Extrusion processing destroys many valuable nutrients in grains. Even granola, a popular "health" food made from grains, is subjected to dry heat and, therefore, extremely indigestible.

Whole grains, such as oatmeal, contain all three parts of the grain: the germ, endosperm and bran. When grains such as wheat or rice are milled or refined, the bran and germ are removed, leaving only the endosperm. The result is a food with fewer vitamins, minerals, fiber, antioxidants and other phytonutrients than the whole grain.

This is why I recommend oatmeal for breakfast every morning. Even though oatmeal is considered mid to high glycemic, oatmeal has low levels of phytic acid and is high in soluble fiber. A morning serving gives you the fast energy you need to start every day and you'll burn it off throughout the morning.

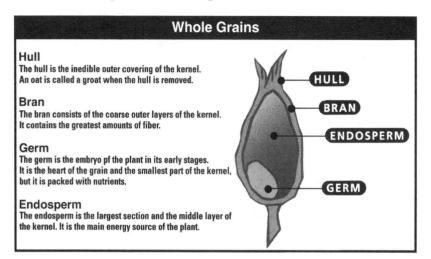

Whole Grains

Hull
The hull is the inedible outer covering of the kernel. An oat is called a groat when the hull is removed.

Bran
The bran consists of the coarse outer layers of the kernel. It contains the greatest amounts of fiber.

Germ
The germ is the embryo pf the plant in its early stages. It is the heart of the grain and the smallest part of the kernel, but it is packed with nutrients.

Endosperm
The endosperm is the largest section and the middle layer of the kernel. It is the main energy source of the plant.

HULL
BRAN
ENDOSPERM
GERM

Whole grains such as oatmeal contain all three parts of the grain: the germ, endosperm and bran. When grains are over processed, the bran and germ are removed, resulting in less nutrients.

 Fiction
We should all follow the new RDA and eat a diet high in grains.

 Fact
Some natural whole grains like oatmeal are healthy, but most people don't do well on a high grain diet. We are omnivores, not herbivores. Unlike herbivores, man only has one stomach. It is difficult to lose fat and build muscle on a diet high in grains.

chapter 15

Fish Can Be "Foul"

Aquaculture (fish farming) is the largest growth industry in the world food economy. In 1985, less than 5% of the world's fish were raised from aquaculture. In 2002, that number has grown to one-third of the world's fish consumption. Nearly all of the rainbow trout, catfish, half the shrimp and half of the salmon consumed in the U.S. are aqua-farmed.

With up to 40,000 fish per pen, each fish spends its life in the equivalent of one bathtub of water. Due to the large number of fish in confined areas, fish farmers must use chemicals to kill bacteria, herbicides to kill vegetation and antibiotics and other chemicals to kill parasites and diseases that would spread rapidly in the holding tanks. This is why farmed fish often contain potentially dangerous levels of antibiotics and chemicals.

Wild salmon develop their pink color from the krill and natural food they eat, but farmed fish are often fed artificial pigments to create this color, as well as vaccines and hormones to enhance growth.

The labels often show a fisherman pulling in a fresh ocean salmon or a fish jumping a waterfall. *We have no idea we're buying farmed fish, because the labels don't tell us.* The fish look the same but they lack the nutrients of wild fish.

No fish or animal manufactures Omega-3 fatty acids; they get them by eating natural foods that contain them and then storing them in their body fat. Wild salmon are an excellent source of Omega-3's but farmed salmon have far less of these essential nutrients.

Independent studies last year conducted in three countries including the U.S. found that farmed fish contained much higher levels of pesticides, including ten times more polychlorinated biphenyls (PCB's) than wild fish. These known toxins affect the central nervous system, lower the immune system and cause cancers in humans.

The aquaculture industry is following in exactly the same direction as the factory livestock farms – bigger fish containing more toxins, hormones and antibiotics, with less nutrients.

The two main protein sources of our early stone age ancestors were fish and meat. We can't go wrong eating ocean white fish like orange roughy. The low fat, high protein content and year round availability make it the best fish to eat when cutting body fat.

Orange Roughy

Calories	76
Fat calories	3
Total fat	0.3 g
Saturated fat	0 g
Cholesterol	—
Sodium	—
Potassium	—
Protein	14.7 g
Iron	—

Serving size 3.5oz.

Orange roughy is an excellent source of low fat, high protein fish.

? Fiction

Most of the fish we buy is caught in the ocean by commercial fishermen.

! Fact

One-third of the fish we buy is aqua-farmed. Each fish is raised in the equivalent of one bathtub of water. Fish farming is the largest growth industry in the world food economy.

chapter 16

Milk & Dairy Products

Got Milk? The Dairy Industry spent $190,000,000 last year to make sure you got it. With over 90% of Americans eating dairy products, apparently the ads are working. Many Americans, however, are coming to the realization that when you consider the facts, dairy products aren't exactly nature's most perfect food. This may help explain why 65% of the world's population doesn't drink milk.

The Stone Agers didn't eat dairy products. They had enough trouble killing wild animals, let alone milking them! Since our early ancestor's diets were high in protein, they didn't have trouble getting enough calcium.

I drink Silk organic calcium and vitamin-enriched soy milk. The dairy industry sued the soy beverages industry for using the word "milk". John Robbins, author of *The Food Revolution*, has an interesting position on this. He says, "for truth in labeling, shouldn't every cow's milk carton say 'cow's milk?' It could be dog milk, or pig milk." Why did humans ever start drinking cow's milk? Even adult cows don't drink cow's milk.

The dairy industry does an outstanding job to convince us otherwise, considering dairy products weren't even considered an essential food group until the 1930's, when the dairy industry began spending big money on research, marketing and advertising to convince us that milk is nature's perfect food.

The big gun for the Dairy Council is *we all need to drink milk to get enough calcium.* The Dairy Bureau says, "For humans to get the calcium they need from food without consuming milk products is extremely difficult."

On the contrary, milk is poorly absorbed by the human digestive system. According to the *American Journal of Clinical Nutrition*, many green vegetables, including Brussels sprouts, mustard greens, broccoli, turnip greens and kale all have calcium absorption rates from 50-64%. The absorption rate for cow's milk is 32%. According to *Bowes and Church's Food Values of Portions Commonly Used*, one cup of milk contains 300 mg. of calcium but only 32% (96 mg) of it is bio-available (what the body can assimilate). You can get this much calcium from just over 1/2 cup tofu made with calcium, 1 1/2 cups cooked broccoli or from 1/2 cup of sesame seeds. In fact, a study by the *American Journal of Epidemiology* concluded "elderly people with the highest dairy consumption actually had double the risk of hip fracture compared to those with the lowest consumption."

Another common problem with dairy products is a sugar called lactose, which is found primarily in dairy products. Lactose intolerance is a condition marked by the inability to digest milk sugar. It is caused by a lack or deficiency of lactase, an enzyme manufactured in the small intestine that splits lactose into simpler forms (glucose and galactose) that can be absorbed by our bodies.

People that don't make enough lactase are "lactose intolerant". When they consume milk or dairy products some or all of the lactose remains undigested and ferments in the colon, resulting in diarrhea, gas, abdominal cramps, nausea and bloating.

Lactose intolerance among adults of different heritage include: Asian 90-100%, Native American 95%, African 65-70%, Hispanic 50-60%, and Caucasian 10%. As you can see, for many of the world's adults, lactose intolerance is a normal condition. Skim milk drinkers face the same risk for health problems due to the chemical make-up of milk, not the fat content.

The Dairy Bureau would have us believe soy milk contains only 3% of the calcium of cow's milk. In fact, most calcium-enriched soy milk contains as much or more calcium as milk.

If the Dairy Bureau gave us the important facts regarding cow's milk vs. soy milk they would include:

- Cow's milk has over eight times as much saturated fat as soy milk.

- Soy milk provides eight times more essential fatty acids as cow's milk.

- Soy beverages are cholesterol free, while cow's milk contains over 30 mg. of cholesterol per cup.

- Soy milk lowers "bad" cholesterol, cow's milk raises it.

- Soy beverages, unlike cow's milk, contain phytoestrogens, which lower heart disease.

- Men who consume one or two servings of soy milk per day are 50% less likely to develop prostate cancer than men who don't.

- Unlike cow's milk, soy milk contains no antibiotics.

I'm not saying you should never eat dairy products. I believe, based on the facts, dairy should be eaten sparingly and is by no means necessary to stay healthy. Give the cow some credit. I put cream in my coffee, and enjoy an occasional fat-free yogurt. Just don't let high profile advertising make you believe dairy should be the foundation of your diet.

Fiction
Milk and dairy products are essential for getting the calcium we need in our daily diets.

Fact
We can get the calcium we need without the fat from natural food and supplements.

chapter 17

Alcohol...Good Or Bad?

Despite the fact that there are hundreds of studies showing why alcohol consumption is harmful to our health, the media jumps all over the few studies that depict alcohol in a positive light. This is unfortunate because it gives drinkers ammunition to rationalize drinking.

The adverse health affects from alcohol far outweigh any benefits. For instance, the anti-oxidants in red grape skins found in red wine are healthy, but the negative health problems caused by the alcohol supercede any health benefits from the grape skins. You don't need to drink alcohol to get anti-oxidants – eat the grapes instead.

Drinking is about the worst thing you can do when trying to lose body fat. Alcohol lowers testosterone, which is just the opposite of what you are trying to achieve. The body processes alcohol much like sugar, and the health effects are even worse.

Alcohol is a very concentrated source of calories (7 calories per gram). When alcohol enters the bloodstream, the liver must reduce or stop its metabolism of fats or carbohydrates and many of its other vital functions to process the alcohol.

Alcohol actually causes a build up of fat in the liver and a decrease in glycogen formation (the body's best fuel source) in the liver and muscles. Alcohol also interferes with processing of niacin, thiamin and B vitamins – all essential for energy production.

Alcohol stimulates appetite and acts as a diuretic, causing loss of precious water – which is needed to lose body fat and gain muscle. If you are overfat to begin with, you gain even more body fat when you drink, because calories from alcohol are burned before stored body fat. Calories from alcohol tend to be stored in the abdomen, thus the term "beer belly".

Drinking light or non-alcoholic beer doesn't reduce calories. Non-alcoholic beer actually has the same calories as regular beer. Drinking a glass of wine before dinner, another glass with dinner and a sweet wine for dessert, will add more than 400 calories to a meal.

The calories in gin, rum, vodka or whiskey depend on the proof, which is twice the percentage of alcohol. For example, 90 proof vodka contains 45% alcohol and 100 proof contains 50% alcohol. The higher the proof, the higher the alcohol content, and the higher the calories.

Think just one drink each night is harmless? One beer every night adds 1,036 additional calories every week, or 15 pounds to your belly every year! A glass of dry wine nightly adds up to about 730 calories every week or about 9 pounds of fat gain each year. It takes an hour on the treadmill just to work off the calories from each glass of wine.

 ## Fiction
A glass of red wine each night is healthy.

 ## Fact
One glass of wine each night adds up to nine pounds of fat gain each year. Alcohol lowers testosterone, slows metabolism, and reduces energy. The adverse health problems far outweigh any benefits.

chapter 18 Genetically Altered Food...Less Nutrients, More Toxins

What do you think of when you hear the term genetically engineered food, GMO or "biotech" food? For years, plant breeders have altered characteristics of plants in order to create improved, desired effects. Oranges could be crossed with other oranges, and apples could be crossed with other apples. Plant breeders were always dealing with other characteristics of the same species.

With modern genetic engineering, however, this isn't the case. *Researchers actually cross species boundaries*, putting genes from one species (or several species) into a second completely different species. Human genes are put into fish, fish genes into tomatoes, and genes from bacteria and rats into broccoli. Many of these engineered fruits and vegetables actually have patents!

Nature hasn't made it easy for cross-species gene splicing. Elephants can't breed with cats, much less humans with fish. It is this crossing of nature's species boundaries that makes the process uniquely powerful and uniquely dangerous. *The same technology that enabled the organism to get into the transgenic organism can enable it to spread and mutate.*

Today, more than half of the processed foods you eat contain byproducts of GMO plants. What are the health consequences of eating this biotech food? The biotech industry would have you believe

GMO foods are fully tested and safe. *The Lancet*, widely recognized as one of the leading medical journals in the world, states candidly, "It is astounding the FDA has not changed their stance on genetically modified food...governments should never have allowed these products into the food chain without insisting on rigorous testing for effects on health."

Our government is trusting companies like Monsanto, the largest biotech giant, to do their own testing. According to the FDA's *Federal Register, Statement of Policy* "Ultimately, it is the food producer who is responsible for assuring safety." Monsanto has been convicted in U.S. courts of a least four major offenses, including providing false information. The EPA ranks Monsanto's factories as having among the largest toxic emissions in the country. It was Monsanto that marketed Agent Orange and PCBs while repeatedly telling us they were safe. *This is a company that could end up controlling most of the food chain for the entire country.*

Genetic engineering essentially moves proteins from one organism to another. In doing this, its possible to transfer allergenic properties to the new food. This already happened in 1996 when soybeans, engineered to include a brazil nut protein, were found to cause a reaction in people allergic to brazil nuts.

Dr. Arpad Pusztai, senior scientist at the Rowett Research Institute in Scotland, is considered a leading world expert on allergies. When he conducted experiments on lab rats, feeding them biotech foods, the rats showed a variety of unexpected and disturbing changes. These changes included smaller livers, hearts and brains, and weakened immune systems.

Dr. John Fagen is a molecular biologist who for more than 20 years was funded by the National Institutes of Health to conduct genetic engineering research. According to Fagen, "Once a gene is inserted into an organism, it can cause unanticipated side effects. A few of these side effects include antibiotic-resistant genes which can be absorbed by humans, the reactivation of dormant or creation of new viruses, new cancers and genetic pollution.

Genetic pollution is when certified organic crops – for example corn – are subject to pollination by GMO corn from neighboring farms. When you consider a 100-acre cornfield throws out over 13 trillion pollen granules, it is no wonder this has already created a problem. Even scarier, is once this happens, there is no way to control further mutations.

Since the advent of cross-species gene splicing we have experienced a dramatic increase of new human diseases including AIDS, West Nile Virus, Ebola, Lyme Disease and Hantavirus, new pathogens that stem from cross-species gene splicing or have come from other species to humans. AIDS is thought to have originated from a virus in chimps and crossed species boundaries to humans. Mad Cow disease is now understood to be the result of a horizontal transfer of an infectious protein that originated in sheep.

We know many of the herbicides (weed killers) developed by the biotech companies for biotech crops pose numerous problems that affect our food supply. Biotech companies develop crops that are resistant to their own brand of herbicides. For instance, the top selling herbicide in the world is Monsanto's Roundup, with over 3 billion in sales last year. Glyphosate, the primary active ingredient in Roundup, has been linked to non-Hodgkin's lymphoma, a serious cancer that affects young people, and the third fastest-growing cancer in the U.S.

Farmers who plant "Roundup ready" biotech seeds can spray this herbicide repeatedly after the crops are planted and growing, without killing the crop. Many biotech crops are resistant to insects because they contain high levels of natural pesticides that insects don't like. Livestock that eat this biotech feed – and people that eat these animals – consume large amounts of these toxic chemicals.

Over half of the foods in supermarkets are genetically altered. Most people are shocked when they learn this. Consumers have no way of knowing they're buying GMO foods, because they aren't labeled. Even the supermarkets often don't know what they're buying. There is only one sure way to avoid eating genetically engineered food in the U.S. and that is to eat organically grown food. No organically grown food is made from transgenic crops. Since it is very hard to find all organic food there are some things to look for when shopping.

Even products that are generally perceived as being "healthy" are often genetically engineered. For example, there are more acres of GMO soybeans being grown than any other transgenic crop.

The majority of all Canola oil sold in the U.S. comes from Canada. Most of Canada's canola (also called rapeseed) crop is genetically engineered. It's almost a certainty that any product containing canola oil includes genetically altered substances.

With potato products, avoid potato starch and potato flour. Most papayas grown in Hawaii are genetically engineered. Most products containing cottonseed oil are genetically altered. Corn is the second largest biotech crop.

For a brand-name shopping guide to non-transgenic foods visit www.safe-food.org. Look for "Organic", "GMO-free" or "Non-GMO" on the labels to be sure the food you are buying is organic.

chapter 19

Labeling Fraud

Most of us actually read the *Nutrition Facts* labels on the food we buy. These labels are helpful when tracking fat grams, sugar and calories. Always check the *Serving Size*, as it is often ridiculously low. Figure the actual amount of the product you'll eat at one meal and the fat and sugar content. Sugar is listed in grams. There are four grams in one teaspoon. Check for sugar substitutes, hydrogenation and preservatives. Look to see if the food is labeled GMO free.

Even though the FDA laws regarding food labeling are a step in the right direction, labels need more information. *The problem is what the nutrition labels don't tell us.* Food processors use labeling laws (or the lack of laws) to conceal, omit and mislead consumers.

Nutrition Facts labels are concealing a hardened killer – trans fat. Most people, even many nutritionists, have never heard of trans fat and the food processing industry would just as soon keep it that way.

Trans fat is made through a heat process, adding hydrogen to liquid vegetable oil in a process called *hydrogenation*. This process forces hydrogen into all the open links of fat's carbon chain during heating. These fats are no longer chemically useful to the body, because humans don't have the digestive power to break the chemical bonds that form during the heating process. These artery clogging, hydrogenated fat globules reduce the body's ability to transport oxygen.

Because this heat process reduces the quantity of antioxidants, the fat is prone to rancidity. Rancid oils are considered risk factors to a host of negative health conditions. These heated fats are known carcinogens.

Trans fat is popular with food processors because it stabilizes food and increases shelf life. The FDA knows trans fat is bad for our cardiovascular systems. Most health experts agree, trans fat is extremely dangerous, especially for people watching their fat intake, diabetics and heart patients.

Walter Willett, a Harvard nutrition researcher, calls trans fat a "triple whammy" – it elevates bad cholesterol, lowers good cholesterol, increases triglycerides and makes blood platelets stickier, increasing the chance of blood clots.

Trans fat, which resembles soap in consistency, is found in over 40,000 products, including chips, cookies, crackers, french fries and salad dressings. It's even found in foods that might seem relatively innocuous, like cereals, low fat soups, rice mixtures and whole wheat breads.

To find the hidden trans fat in food, look for the word "hydrogenated" on the nutrition label. If you find this word, subtract the saturated fat content from the total fat content. The fat remaining is probably trans fat .

Although this calls for fast action, the FDA still doesn't require the labeling of trans fat, although legislation is supposedly in the works. Lawrence Bachorik, a head FDA official, says "We have lost some employees and have been focusing on food safety initiatives." The FDA's lack of urgency is typical of their attitude regarding diet and health issues.

A cost-benefit done in 1999 estimated that labeling trans fat would save $3-8 billion annually in averted heart disease costs, and save 2000-5000 lives each year. The Center for Science in the Public Interest, which promotes nutrition labels, estimates labeling trans fat could prevent up to 17,000 new cases of coronary artery disease each year. According to the Center's spokeswoman, "If this was an infectious disease, the government would be on top of it in minutes."

Nutrition labels also don't tell us the glycemic index of the food we're buying. As more of us begin to realize how important the glycemic index is, especially when trying to lose body fat, healthy food distributors will respond by testing and listing it on food labels.

CURRENT LABELING

Nutrition Facts

Serving Size:1

Amount Per Serving

Calories 200 Calories from fat 80

	%Daily Value*
Total Fat 9g	14%
Saturated Fat 3g	15%
Polyunsaturated Fat 1g	
Monounsaturated Fat 4g	
Cholesterol 0mg	0%
Sodium 33mg	4%
Total Carbohydrate 27g	9%
Dietary Fiber 1g	
Sugars Less than 1g	
Protein 4g	

Vitamin A 0%	Vitamin C 0%
Calcium 2%	Iron 8%

*Percent Daily Values are based on a 2,000 calorie diet. Your daily values may be higher or lower depending on your calorie needs:

Calories:		2,000	2,500
Total Fat	Less than	65g	80g
Sat Fat	Less than	20g	25g
Cholesterol	Less than	300mg	300mg
Sodium	Less than	2400mg	2400mg
Total Carbohydrate		300g	375g
Dietary Fiber		25g	30g

MADE FROM: UNBLEACHED ENRICHED WHEAT FLOUR (FLOUR, NIACIN, REDUCED IRON, THIAMIN MONONITRATE (VITAMIN B1), RIOFLAVIN (VITAMIN B2), FOLIC ACID), NONFAT MILK, **PARTIALLY HYDROGENATED VEGETABLE SHORTENING** (SOYBEAN AND OR COTTONSEED AND/OR CANOL...)

Under current labeling, the best clue that trans fat lurks is the word "hydrogenated"

PROPOSED LABELING

Under one proposed label, trans fat would be lumped in with saturated fat. The precise breakdown would be explained with an asterisk. Some nutritionists argue this would be the clearest approach, because many people already are trying to avoid saturated fat, but don't realize how much trans fat they're eating.

Nutrition Facts

Serving Size:1 Tsbp (14g)
Servings Per Container 32

Amount Per Serving

Calories 100	Calories from fat 100	
	%Daily Value*	
Total Fat 9g	11g	17%
Saturated Fat**	11g	20%
Cholesterol	0mg	0%
Sodium	115mg	5%
Total Carbohydrate	0g	0%
Protein 0g		

Vitamin A 6%

Not a significant source of dietary fiber, sugars vitamin C, calcium and iron.

*Percent Daily Values are based on a 2,000 calorie diet. Your daily values may be higher or lower depending on your calorie needs:

**Includes 6g trans fat.

In Europe, this is already done by many food distributors.

Many of us read labels to tell us if the meat (chicken, turkey, beef, etc.) and eggs we buy are "range fed". According to Allen Shainsky, author of *Rocky the Chicken*, "When it comes to the words natural or free range – federal law is and always was toothless. It doesn't guarantee a thing. Poultry companies use free range strictly as a marketing gimmick. Legally, the phrase means nothing. There is no law or regulation defining free range. Natural is another meaningless term – by USDA's standards a Burger King Whopper is natural."

More Labeling Deception – Fat Free Fraud

Another misleading, although legal, labeling ploy is "fat free" claims commonly found on processed meat. When following a reduced fat, high protein diet, this sounds great – we get all that protein without much fat. A closer look reveals the ugly truth. Although "97% fat free" is accurate by the letter of the law (i.e., a 28 gram slice of meat containing 1 gram of fat = 3% fat by weight = 97% fat free), it is misleading regarding true nutrient content. If we check the Nutrition Facts box and do some quick division, dividing fat calories by total calories, we'll see 30% of the calories are from fat!

The other ingredients are fillers such as water injected into the meat during processing. While these cheap fillers add bulk, weight and moisture to the meat, they don't add calories. So a 28-gram slice of luncheon meat could end up containing only 6 grams of protein. Figuring 4 calories per gram, the protein provides 20 calories, and at 9 calories per gram the fat adds 9 calories, for total calorie count of 29 and a fat-calorie percentage of over 30%. Food with 30% of calories from fat is not low fat!

When buying turkey or chicken, don't buy "ground lean" de-boned products. When processors mechanically separate the meat from the bones they often package about every part of the bird except the organs, which they have to label. This includes the skin, the tendons, and connective tissues.

If you compare a four ounce chunk of fresh white meat turkey with ground turkey you'll see the difference. Fresh turkey contains 36 grams of protein and is about 60% water by weight. Processed turkey typically contains about 18 grams of protein and is 75% water by weight. It's more profitable to sell water than protein. Fresh turkey breast is about 18% calories from fat compared to processed turkey which is about 50% calories from fat. A fresh 4-ounce slice of turkey breast has about 90 milligrams of sodium. Most processed meat is full of sodium – up to 1,200 milligrams per 4-ounce serving.

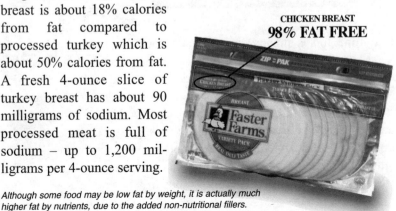

CHICKEN BREAST
98% FAT FREE

Although some food may be low fat by weight, it is actually much higher fat by nutrients, due to the added non-nutritional fillers.

Certified Organic Labeling

The new USDA Organic Foods Production Act now requires foods touted as "organic" to meet certain guidelines. In the past, private certifying agencies and state regulations allowed crops fertilized with sewage sludge, bio-engineered and irradiated foods to be labeled as "organic". Products that contained only small amounts of organic food could also be labeled "organic".

These new labeling requirements apply to raw, fresh products and processed foods that contain organic ingredients. The USDA has created four organic categories. *Foods* labeled "100% organic" must contain only organically produced ingredients. *Products* labeled "organic" must consist of at least 95% organically produced ingredients. The *"made with organic ingredients"* category includes processed products that contain at least 70% organic ingredients and list up to 3 of the organic ingredients or food groups on the principal display panel. *Processed products* that contain less than 70% organic ingredients cannot use the term "organic" on the principal display panel.

These new labeling guidelines are a step in the right direction but the problem remains; the USDA has failed to enforce labeling laws in the past and has no budget to do so in the future. The terms "natural, free-range, no drugs or growth hormones used, and sustainable harvested" are misleading labeling tactics, which mean nothing. Look for the USDA ORGANIC label to be sure the food is actually organic.

❓ Fiction

Food nutrition labels tell us everything we need to know about the food we buy in order to eat healthy.

❗ Fact

Food nutrition labels are often misleading because food processors don't list the amount of transfat, and don't tell us if foods are genetically modified, "natural" or "USDA Organic". Processors can label food low fat using weight, not calories.

PART

4

Eating Right To Lose Body Fat

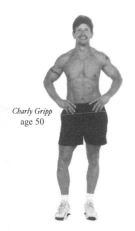

Charly Gripp
age 50

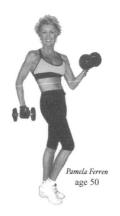

Pamela Ferren
age 50

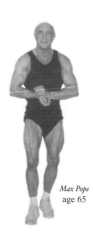

Max Pope
age 65

chapter 20

Diet Is As Important As Exercise

Most health experts agree proper diet accounts for at least 75% of the total fitness program, exercise is about 20% and supplementation is about 5%. The problem is, many disagree on what type of diet is the healthiest.

The government's food pyramid advises us to eat between six and eleven servings of cereal grains daily and two to three servings of dairy foods. Nutritional authorities such as Dr. Dean Ornish encourage us to lower dietary fat to less than 10% of calories and eat plenty of whole grains and legumes. Nutritional expert Dr. Neal Barnard advises us to eliminate all animal products from our diets. In stark contrast, the popular Atkins Diet advises us to dramatically reduce carbs and eat all the fat we want. Whom should we believe?

The *Muscle & Longevity* diet is similar to the way our early ancestors ate, the way we're genetically programmed to eat for optimal health and longevity. It is through this balanced diet with high intensity, short duration exercise and prolonged high-intensity training that we get – and stay – fit. Not only do people on my program have better physiques and look healthier – they *are* healthier!

The best combination of daily calories for most people to stay fit and healthy is 40-45% protein, 40-45% carbohydrates, and 15-20% good fat. The protein reduces appetite while supplying essential amino acids for muscle growth. The mid-low glycemic carbohydrates supply energy throughout the day, and the good fat supplies the essential fatty acids we need.

Eat Enough Protein

Have you ever heard anyone say "We can get all the protein we need from a normal diet?" The question is "need for what?" There's a huge difference between just surviving and building lean muscle.

To sustain life we need about 36 grams of protein per 100 pounds of body weight. Recent research has proven five times this much may be required to obtain maximum increases in strength and lean mass. The average daily caloric intake of protein in the U.S. is only 15.5%. Our early ancestors ate three times this much protein. *The same high protein diet is essential to grow muscle and keep the brain sharp.*

Protein contains the amino acids our bodies need to grow and repair damaged tissue from weight lifting. Plus, these amino acids provide optimal levels of dopamine and serotonin levels to the brain, necessary for mental, emotional and sexual well-being.

Our bodies can assimilate about 40 grams of protein every four hours, but can't stockpile amino acids; any extra is just passed out in our urine. If we're not eating protein every few hours, our supply of amino acids will diminish, and those in the tissues are sucked out, resulting in a net loss of tissue protein.

When we reduce calories to lose body fat, we need even more protein. *Protein is the primary nutrient for facilitating muscle hypertrophy, or growth.* If we don't get protein every few hours, our bodies can easily regress into a catabolic state. When this happens, the starvation mechanism is activated and our bodies actually start cannibalizing our hard-earned muscle, leaving our fat stores untouched!

Protein has more vagus nerve-stimulating ability than carbohydrates or glucose. Stimulating the vagus nerve signals us to stop eating. Protein stabilizes our insulin and energy levels. Without it, our blood sugar would fluctuate all day, causing "highs" and "lows", as well as food cravings. This is why *protein is the foundation of a healthy diet.*

Most of us, especially women, don't eat enough protein. Eating a few pieces of chicken at night doesn't give us adequate protein throughout the day. Unfortunately, muscle growth takes place over a period of days, not right after we train. This is why we should eat protein at every meal and supplement protein between meals.

Some people don't digest animal protein well. Don't become a vegetarian – fix the digestion problem. Those of us that have a hard time digesting meat should not avoid it on those grounds any more than a poorly tuned car should avoid high-octane gasoline. Use hydrochloric acid supplements, herbal bitters and pancreatic enzymes to help aid digestion. A "tuned up" digestive system enables our bodies to burn the fuel it was meant to burn.

The WHO (World Health Organization) set the minimum protein intake at about 1/3 gram of protein per pound of body weight (see chart below). Studies show weight lifters need at least one gram (or more) of protein for every pound of body weight.

Ideal Weight	Daily Protein Suggestions			
	Minimum	**Medium**	**Typical**	**Bodybuilder**
	0.34g/lb.	0.5g/lb.	1g/lb.	1.3g/lb.
80 lbs.	27g	40g	80g	104g
100 lbs.	34g	50g	100g	130g
120 lbs.	41g	60g	120g	156g
140 lbs.	48g	70g	140g	182g
160 lbs.	54g	80g	160g	208g
180 lbs.	61g	90g	180g	234g
200 lbs.	68g	100g	200g	260g
220 lbs.	75g	110g	220g	286g

Weight lifters need more protein, at least 1-1.5 grams for each pound of body weight.

According to a strength and health report issued by Penn State Center for Medicine, "There is overwhelming data indicating that for those athletes engaged in intense and regular endurance or strength training, the RDA for protein is sub-optimal." The Nutrition for Sport and Exercise Dept. of University of Colorado agrees saying, "The RDA for protein would seem insufficient for those persons who are developing muscular mass and strength using a heavy resistance training program." These are just a few of hundreds of recent studies done by health and athletic organizations around the world.

Some think it is unhealthy to eat a high protein diet. This notion is one of the most pervasive nutritional myths remaining today. It dates back to an experiment years ago that demonstrated rodents on high protein diets developed a serious kidney condition known as nephrocalcinosis. Nephrocalcinosis has never been detected in humans. Both epidemiological and clinical observations prove quite conclusively that even extraordinarily high amounts of protein don't result in kidney or liver dysfunction in healthy people. (Individuals with existing liver, kidney or pancreatic disease need to monitor protein intake as directed by their physician.)

Lean animal protein actually helps protect the heart by raising protective HDL (good) cholesterol levels. Being afraid of protein is like being afraid of love. It's good for you, and life without it isn't what it should be!

? **Fiction**
If you just exercise, you'll lose body fat.

! **Fact**
Exercise is important, but proper diet is 75% of any successful fat-loss program.

chapter 21

Reduce High Glycemic Carbohydrates To Achieve Ketosis

C arbohydrates (carbs) are the sugars (simple and complex) found in foods like fruits, vegetables, tubers, grains, breads, pastas, rolls, cookies, cakes, candies, juices and sodas. As I discussed earlier, carbs come in two varieties: paleocarbs (fruits and vegetables), the kind mankind has consumed for millions of years, and neocarbs, those grain legume based, high glycemic refined carbs that have developed since the Industrial Revolution.

Ketosis (when the body starts burning stored fat for energy) gets its name from a group of three substances called ketone bodies, which are formed during digestion of low-glycemic carbs. Our bodies use these ketones safely and effectively for energy. Ketone bodies are special fat-like compounds, which are water-soluble. They are used for energy by most of our body tissues, except the liver. They are an ideal energy source to achieve increased metabolism.

When cutting body fat, it's essential to reduce our consumption of neocarbs and high glycemic carbs. Reducing these types of carbs helps us achieve ketosis rapidly. Although we should reduce our intake of these calorie-dense, high glycemic carbs, we should eat no more than 40% of our daily calories from mid and low-glycemic carbs. It is essential to eat these low and mid glycemic carbs because carbohydrates equal glycogen. Glycogen is stored in the liver and muscles and converted into fuel as the muscles need it for high intensity exercise like weight lifting. Low glycemic foods are especially good to eat before exercising, because they enter the bloodstream slowly and provide long term energy.

Carbs are the only food that can be used for anaerobic energy for weight lifting. Carbs are the most efficient fuel for aerobic exercise because carbs produce energy three times faster than fat and require less oxygen to do so. At more intense levels of aerobic exercise, carbs are utilized nearly exclusively for an energy source.

Keeping a steady flow of low glycemic carbs is essential for our high intensity, short duration and prolonged cardio exercise training. It is through this synergistic program that ketosis is achieved and fat stores are tapped while building muscle. Low glycemic foods include vegetables such as broccoli, squash, green beans, spinach, asparagus, Brussels sprouts, and cabbage.

Our early ancestors ate fruit, but the fruit was much different than today's "chemically enhanced" super fruits. Early man ate smaller fruits with less fructose, and usually only in the summer months. Most fruits are healthy, *but when reducing body fat, fructose (sugar) should be eaten in limited amounts*. A half grapefruit, apple or pear with breakfast is adequate. We're getting the vitamins we need from supplements, without the sugar and calories.

Eating too many high and mid glycemic carbs can cause the body to choose sugar, as opposed to fat, as its primary fuel source for everyday activity. Fat refers to not only the fat we eat, but stored body fat as well.

Some people believe that calorie restriction (CR) induced ketosis is unhealthy. Although ketosis isn't recommended for type 1 diabetics, those with kidney failure,

Highly Glycemic Foods		Moderately Glycemic Foods		Low Glycemic Foods	
Glucose	100	Orange Juice	57	Apple	36
Baked Potato	85	White Rice	56	Pear	34
Corn Flakes	84	Popcorn	55	Skim Milk	32
Cheerios	74	Corn	55	Green Beans	30
Graham Crakers	74	Brown Rice	55	Lentils	29
Honey	73	Sweet Potato	54	Kidney Beans	27
Watermelon	72	(Ripe) Banana	50	Grapefruit	25
White Bread/Bagel	70-72	Orange	43	Barley	25
Table Sugar	65	Apple Juice	41		
Raisins	64				

or for pregnant women, long term research has proven the rest of us can do just fine in ketosis, even for years.

Other Benefits From Ketosis

Short-term ketogenic dieting not only reduces body fat, but is also proven to slow down the aging process. A genetic study published in the August 1999 issue of *Science* found that calorie reduction (CR), blocked 84% of the gene activity that triggers cellular aging in animals. Other genes controlling beneficial processes such as response to overheating, DNA repair and oxidative stress, doubled in activity after a CR eating plan.

In a study reported in the June 1997 issue of the *FASB Journal*, rats on a CR diet showed prevention of age-related muscle fiber loss and decreased muscle mitochondrial damage due to oxidation effects. The lab rats began the diet at the human equivalent of middle age. Other studies started in 1972 at UCLA by pathologist Roy Walford have showed CR slowed aging in a wide variety of species including rats, worms, and flies.

Numerous studies have shown animals and humans on a ketogenic diet actually increase muscle size, muscle endurance, and muscle strength as long as they lift weights or do resistance exercises. I've found I can gain muscle for about three months in ketosis, and then I start losing muscle. I also believe it is important to supplement vitamins and minerals during ketosis to maintain health and energy levels.

In studies, animals have shown the same beneficial results with just a 10% CR when combined with resistance training as with a 30% CR without training. Another study that started in 1987 at the National Institute of Aging and the University of Wisconsin has shown that rhesus and squirrel monkeys (man's closest relatives) that are eating 30% fewer calories than other monkeys are aging slower. The monkeys also process glucose better, show decreased insulin sensitivity and show less incidence of cancer.

For most of us, CR induced ketosis is a wonderful thing. CR helps many people lose body fat who otherwise cannot. You can determine if you're in ketosis, and at what level, using ketone strips which can be purchased at drug stores. These strips measure the amount of ketones you pass in your urine.

Don't Severely Restrict Carbs

There is a big difference between reducing high and mid glycemic carbs and severely restricting all carbohydrates like some popular low carbohydrate diets. Many "diet experts" suggest that if we just do away with those dreaded carbs, we'll lose weight without exercising.

Any diet that severely restricts carbohydrates will always result in the rapid depletion of muscle glycogen, liver glycogen and water, all essential for proper biochemical reactions to exercise properly. The *Muscle & Longevity* program requires glycogen for the energy we must have to build muscle, reduce body fat, and live healthy lives.

For most people, the negative health effects of severe carb restriction far outweigh the advantages. These carbohydrate depletion diets include *Protein Power, Carbohydrate Addict's Diet* and *Dr. Atkin's New Diet Revolution*.

Just how extreme is the Atkins diet? The typical American diet averages about 2 grams of carbs per pound of body weight each day or 300 grams for a 150-pound person. The Atkins diet consists of about *20 grams daily* the first two weeks, and then increases to about 40 grams daily.

Dr. Atkins believes that when carbohydrates are severely restricted and we eliminate glycogen (glucose), our main energy source, the results are low blood sugar levels. This causes our bodies to produce less insulin so our cells don't get the energy they need to live. The body is then forced to turn to stored body fat by breaking down fat molecules into glycerin and fatty acids. These fatty acids are then processed into simple fatty acids, which become energy.

If everything actually worked liked this you'd be burning body fat, and since you're not eating carbohydrates, you wouldn't be storing any body fat. **What Dr. Atkins doesn't tell you is that fat isn't the only source of energy your body uses when severely cutting carbohydrates**. Your body actually starts cannibalizing hard earned muscle because muscle burns calories and fat doesn't. The next thing your body does is begin lowering your metabolism to conserve energy. The more muscle you lose, the lower your metabolism drops. This is exactly the opposite of what you want to achieve!

As a result, Atkin's dieters actually *achieve weight loss mostly from water and muscle loss, not fat*. The water loss occurs because starchy foods are broken down in the body and stored with water (each gram of glycogen stored in muscle tissue also stores about 3 grams of water with it). So the resulting weight loss usually includes between seven and ten pounds of water loss within the first few weeks on the diet. Water is something we need to build muscle.

Inadequate carbs result in low liver and glycogen supplies (the storage form of glucose). This dramatically reduces the rate that dieters can convert fat and protein to glucose. The results are lethargy, depression, decreased sexual drive, chronic fatigue, insomnia, frequent infections and the inability to exercise properly. The scarcity of dietary fiber in this diet is linked to many cancers. This type of high fat, low carb diet often leads to cardiovascular disease. Atkins himself recently had heart trouble despite his assurance that it is not diet related. On the *Muscle & Longevity* Program, you can eat all the low glycemic carbs you want for slow release energy and adequate fiber.

❓ Fiction

We should severely restrict eating carbohydrates to lose body fat.

❗ Fact

We should eat a balanced diet of low-glycemic carbohydrates, protein and "smart" fat to achieve healthy ketosis.

chapter 22

Drink Enough Water

Next to oxygen, water is the most important element the body needs to survive. Without water, we can die in three days. Most of us are chronically dehydrated and 37% of us have a thirst-mechanism so weak that it is often mistaken for hunger.

Our bodies are mostly water; 75% of our brains are water, our blood is 82% water, and even our bones are 25% water. Young people hold more water than older people do and females hold more water than males. *As incredible as it may seem, water is the most important catalyst in the metabolism of fats.*

Adequate water is essential to maintain elevated metabolism. A decrease in water intake can cause fat deposits to increase, while an increase in water intake actually reduces fat deposits and suppresses the appetite naturally. As our body senses a decrease in the availability of fluid, our hormonal systems will actually alter the fluid balance and cause our body to retain as much water as possible.

The body sees dehydration as a threat to survival and holds onto every precious drop, even storing water in extra cellular spaces (outside the cells). Along with fluid retention, edema may occur, causing obesity, swollen feet, legs, hands and face. We can thank our paleolithic ancestors for this genetic trait that helped them survive droughts.

When we don't drink enough water, our bodies aren't able to filter the blood properly, resulting in a metabolic overload on the liver. One of the liver's primary functions is to metabolize stored fat into usable energy for the body. When the liver has to do some of the kidneys' work, such as detoxify contaminated water, it can't operate to its fullest capacity. As a result, the liver metabolizes less fat, resulting in more stored body fat.

Water is the main component of blood, which transports nutrients and wastes. A lack of it can cause fats and other toxins that should be passed, to remain in our body, This includes the dimpled fat commonly referred to as cellulite. People on high protein diets require adequate water in order to rid the body of excess nitrogen compounds (a bi-product of protein breakdown) that are free floating in the body. When we're exercising and burning fat, we have a lot more metabolized fat and other toxins to get rid of. We need adequate water to flush out this waste.

An average person should consume approximately 96 ounces or three quarts of water each day. An active or athletic person needs considerably more (up to 1 to 1 1/2 gallons per day). This is because they sweat more, thereby losing more water through the evaporative process. Fit people actually sweat faster and more than unfit people because their "cooling" systems are more effective.

Don't make the mistake of drinking coffee, tea, fruit juice or even wine or beer, in place of water. Even though recent studies show some of the water in these drinks and food are absorbed, it still isn't as effective as pure water. The kidneys cannot function as efficient on this "contaminated" water because it doesn't have the same chemical properties as water. Alcohol, soft drinks and fruit juice (to a lesser degree) contain too much sugar, which inhibits the absorption of water.

Water gives muscle the natural ability to contract by preventing dehydration. *If we dehydrate a muscle by only 3%, we cause a 10 % loss of contractile strength and a 8% loss of speed. Even mild dehydration will slow our metabolism as much as 3% , cause fuzzy short term memory and cause difficulty focusing our eyes.*

Water is essential when reducing calories. Just one glass stops midnight hunger pangs for most people. Lack of water is the leading cause of daytime fatigue. Research has proven adequate water eases back and joint pain for 80% of sufferers, decreases risk of colon cancer by 50%, breast cancer by 80%, and bladder cancer by 50%.

If we lose enough water to become dehydrated, we also lose precious electrolytes which keep the body in fluid balance, regulate body temperature and process many biochemical reactions. When this happens, muscles cramp, dizziness and weakness occur and perspiration no longer cools us. Rising core temperature causes heat cramps, heat exhaustion, heat stroke and eventually death.

Overfat people, especially women, require more water than normal. Recent studies have shown that overfat individuals who did nothing more than increase their water intake to 96 oz. or more per day lost an average of 7-12 pounds of weight in one year. Water helps to prevent the sagging skin that often follows weight loss. Shrinking cells are buoyed by water, which helps plump and tighten the skin. The overfat person needs one additional glass for every 25 pounds of excess body fat.

When we exercise hard, we produce enough heat to evaporate two quarts of water per hour! We should drink water even when we're not thirsty. Don't worry about drinking too much water – it's impossible, because the body simply passes it as urine or sweat. We lose an average of 28-40 ounces each day in breath and perspiration and 20-53 ounces in urine.

Diuretics

Diuretics offer a temporary and unhealthy solution for weight loss. They force out stored water along with essential nutrients, stripping the body of precious minerals. This can rapidly create a serious electrolyte imbalance. Diuretics often cause constipation by draining water in the colon in order to distribute it throughout our body to make up for the shortages. When constipation occurs from lack of water, most people experience a weight loss plateau. The best way to overcome the problem of constipation and water retention is to give the body what it needs – plenty of water!

Water Retention-Sodium

People who have a problem with water retention often consume too much salt/sodium and don't drink enough water. Humans will tolerate only a certain amount of sodium. People in normal health should consume no more than 2000 milligrams of sodium a day. Two thousand milligrams is the equivalent of one teaspoon of salt. One large dill pickle has about 720 milligrams of sodium.

The more sodium we eat, the more water we need to dilute it. If we don't drink enough water after high sodium foods, our bodies pull water from the intestines to dilute the extra sodium. The water is stored in extra-cellular spaces, making us look overfat. Getting rid of excess sodium is easy – drink more water.

If you have a problem with water retention, take the salt shaker off the dining table and select brands that are lowest in sodium, disodium phosphate or monosodium glutamate (they're just as bad). Watch for sodium in softened water, bottled water, medications, antacids and salted foods like pretzels and many processed foods. Caffeine has a diuretic effect and diet soda contains sodium, which also contributes to water retention.

Sports Drinks

Many of the sports drinks found at the gym contain thermogenics, sugar, glucose or sugar substitutes which we should avoid. Some athletes, like distance runners, require a steady trickle of glucose for maintaining energy. When trying to achieve ketosis, however, these drinks cause blood insulin to rise, and insulin inhibits fat burning.

The labels on these drinks often say "electrolytes added". Any mineral can be an electrolyte, but the main ones include sodium, potassium and chloride. These are the common minerals added to most sports drinks. The labels could just say "added minerals", but it loses some marketing punch (no pun intended).

Most sports drinks contain the same amount of sodium and potassium as a glass of soy milk and a bite of banana. Unless we're competing in a marathon or triathlon, we don't lose many electrolytes. *It's the replacement of water that's important.*

The simplest, healthiest, and most effective sports drinks can be made simply by blending a banana in a few quarts of water. This will supply the necessary water, sugar (glucose and fructose) and electrolytic minerals while providing adequate vitamins and enzymes to properly metabolize them.

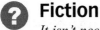

Fiction
It isn't necessary to drink more water when "cutting".

Fact
We need to increase water intake on a fat-to-muscle program to elevate metabolism, deliver nutrients to muscles and remove toxins from body.

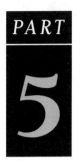

PART
5

Exercising After Middle Age

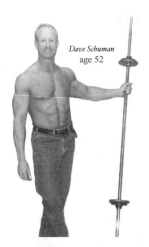

Dave Schuman
age 52

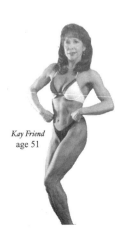

Kay Friend
age 51

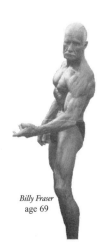

Billy Fraser
age 69

chapter 23

We Can Gain Muscle At Any Age

Modern research has proven weight training is essential to staying healthy as we age. What used to be the "black sheep" of athletics is now the very foundation of all athletic sports. Although actually turning fat into muscle isn't possible, most people will make a fat-to-muscle transition on the *Muscle & Longevity* Program.

Until recently, most scientists believed that once we reached middle age, our chances of making significant muscle gains were slim. About the most we could hope for was to firm up and get stronger.

This dogma was dismissed when studies conducted by Tufts University in Boston demonstrated conclusively that we can make muscular gains at any age. Even people over age 90 made significant gains with strength, improving from 30-100% in just 90 days.

Weight training is the only proven way to maintain muscle mass and strength with age. Weight training stimulates our bodies (both women and men) to produce hormones such as free testosterone and human growth hormone necessary for new muscle growth. It also improves the efficiency with which cells use testosterone.

Chapter 24 Strength Training For Patients With Heart Disease

S trength training has always played second fiddle to aerobics and flexibility exercises – especially for people with heart problems or recent heart surgery. Physicians warned that physical activity, especially weight training, would burden already overloaded hearts.

New studies by an expert panel of scientists sponsored by the American Heart Association finally puts this type of thinking to rest. This committee has advised doctors to recommend strength training in conjunction with aerobics for not only older healthy patients, but for patients with heart disease, including some patients who suffered recent heart attacks. Of course, any such activity should be closely monitored and supervised by experienced health care professionals.

A recent study by Dr. Kerry Bernard and colleagues from the River Cities Cardiology Clinic in Indiana found that adding strength training to an exercise program in heart failure patients increased their strength an average of 26%. Patients had a better quality of life without worsening their medical conditions.

Doctors now realize that weight training is essential for preventing or controlling diabetes (a major risk factor for heart disease), high cholesterol and high blood pressure. Both aerobic and weight lifting strengthen the heart muscle, helping it work more efficiently.

Experts have long agreed that aerobic exercise helps lower systolic and diastolic blood pressure. Recent research by Dr. George Kelly, a researcher in the department of kinesiology and physical education at Northern Illinois University, now indicates a regular program of weight lifting actually lowers a person's blood pressure at rest as well.

Fiction

If you suffer from heart disease, you shouldn't exercise.

Fact

Doctors now recommend lifting weights and aerobics for older healthy patients and patients with heart disease, including patients who have suffered recent heart attacks.

chapter 25

Baby Boomers Have Advantages and Disadvantages

Middle aged athletes have many advantages over our younger counterparts. Heart rate and time to fatigue is not significantly different between 20 and 50 years of age. We are usually more patient (you don't see the positive effects from weight training overnight). We understand our bodies better than young people. We know it takes hard work to succeed at anything and we often have the financial resources for the best supplements, gyms and trainers. More good news is that we're blessed with a wide variety of new supplements that help slow down the aging process and build muscle.

How many times have you heard someone say, "I'm getting older and my metabolism is slowing down?" Just because we're older doesn't mean our metabolism should be slower, unless we're in poor physical shape. The resting basil metabolic rate (BMR) of a 20-year-old male weighing 154 pounds compared to a 60-year-old male weighing the same is 1,755 vs. 1,692 respectively – only 63 fewer calories.

If I've made a believer out of you and you're ready to hit the gym, you need to follow a few simple rules to stay healthy and prevent injury. Most middle age people are overfat, don't heal as fast, often have old injuries, have lower testosterone and growth hormone levels, have less fast twitch fibers and often have higher blood pressure.

With proper exercise, adequate sleep, proper diet and supplements, older folks will make significant gains, but probably slower than our younger counterparts. We especially need to make sure we get more rest between workouts and take the proper supplements to help our bodies recover.

Most muscle groups recover within 24 hours. Larger muscles, like legs, usually recover within 36 hours. The rule of thumb is always *listen to your body*. If a muscle group is still sore don't work it until it recovers. If you start feeling run-down, take a day or two off. You'll come back feeling strong and ready to attack the weights.

Fiction
Middle age athletes' tire much faster than younger athletes.

Fact
Middle aged athletes heart rate and time to fatigue is about the same as a 20 year old.

chapter 26

Don't Stretch Like Young People

Flexibility is an important component of overall fitness. "Short" muscle fibers that are sticking together lack flexibility. These muscles perform less effectively and can lead to nerve pain and injury. Contrary to popular belief, weight training does not reduce flexibility when done properly.

Most people actually increase flexibility following the *Muscle & Longevity* program by stretching *during* workouts instead of before or after. Unless you're into yoga or are an elite athlete, "conventional" stretching sessions do very little to improve flexibility and are difficult, time consuming and often dangerous. This probably contradicts everything you've heard about doing a short aerobic "warm-up" and stretching before weight lifting.

There are two ways flexibility can be improved: through *mechanical* stretching of the muscles, tendons and ligaments, and through *resetting neural regulation* of muscular length. Mechanical stretching can be compared to stretching a rubber band to a greater length using brute force.

Unless you are ten years old, pregnant, or take daily injections of the hormone relaxin, *mechanical* stretching is out (unless you're into pain and injury). This is because adult connective tissue is mostly scar tissue. The older you are, the more scar tissue you have and the less flexible you are. This means you are more susceptible to injury from stretching.

Resetting the set point for the length of our muscles is the safe way to increase flexibility. The central nervous system sets a "favorite" length for a muscle based on the length it remembers best either from *extensive* or *intensive* learning. Extensive learning is when your body memorizes something when you keep repeating it.

Intensive learning occurs when a stimulus has made a strong impression on you. For instance, a caller informs you that you've just won the lottery, and you remember the lucky number. *Weight training is an extremely strong intensive learning stimulus.* When you utilize *time & resistance* weight training, it makes a regular 20-minute stretching session look tame by comparison.

Middle aged or older people who warm-up with a few minutes of aerobic exercise before stretching are asking for trouble. They're not warm enough. This conventional type stretching session is neither extensive nor intensive. For the average weight lifter, it really has little or no effect on the nervous system. After 30 deep leg presses, your quad and hamstring lengths will be set based on the range of motion of the leg presses, not the stretches.

The *Muscle & Longevity* program incorporates stretching the individual muscle groups you are training *before and during sets*. If you aren't warmed up, cold muscles don't stretch as well, are more prone to injury, are less efficient at burning fat and aren't getting the blood supply to operate at maximum capacity.

When you warm up individual muscle groups using light-weight and high reps, your heart pumps more blood, the muscles fill with blood, the capillaries become dilated and the entire nervous system becomes sharper. Stretches for the specific muscle groups you're working are held at least 15-20 seconds and never forced. Following this warm-up and stretching technique enables you to add muscle, increase flexibility and reduces the chance of injury.

❓ Fiction
Always warm up and stretch before lifting weights.

❗ Fact
Middle aged and older athletes should use light weight to warm up the muscle group targeted, and stretch between, during and after sets.

chapter 27

Muscle Soreness & Icing

If I'm not sore the day after lifting, I know I didn't push myself hard enough. This delayed muscle soreness (DMS) is caused by damage to the cellular membrane or small micro-tears from lifting. The more our muscles become adapted to lifting, the less DMS we'll experience.

Once the damage has occurred to the muscle, the body starts "rebuilding" the muscle by releasing metabolites and hormones that facilitate repair and growth. The bad news is, it takes about 24 hours to replenish glycogen supplies, 1-2 hours to remove lactic acid and up to 3 days or longer to rebuild the damaged muscle tissue. The fatigued muscles need time to recuperate.

The good news is, we rebuild the damaged muscles stronger than before! After all, our muscles don't know we're lifting weights. We're still programmed to survive 40,000 years ago. Our brains telling our muscles we're building a cave or hauling a mammoth carcass back to the clan. Our bodies are building more lean muscle mass to get stronger to survive.

Important steps for optimal muscle recovery from DMS include proper diet; supplements, (vitamin-minerals with anti-oxidants); lots of water to help flush the toxins from the body, lots of sleep; and stretching during weight lifting sessions.

Although there is no scientific explanation as to the exact benefits of massage therapy, I recommend regular massages. Relaxed muscle fibers work better than tight (short) fibers which can lead to injury.

Icing Injured Muscles

Nearly everyone who exercises suffers at one time or another from pulled muscles, sprains or tendonitis. Most of us know the therapeutic value of icing injuries, but few really know the most effective way to ice.

Dr. Domhnall MacAuley, a muscle therapeutic specialist at the University of Ulster in Northern Ireland, has carried out extensive comprehensive scientific studies on icing injuries. Here's his advice on the subject.

"Ice is the best, cheapest and most effective anti-inflammatory." After a strain, inflammation usually follows. Blood vessels at the injury site expand, which cause pain, swelling and the accumulation of fluid, or edema. According to MacAuley, the application of ice can reduce swelling, curbing pain.

His research shows that melting ice water applied through a wet towel for repeated periods of ten minutes is most effective. Used repeatedly, rather than continuously, ice applications help sustain reduced muscle temperatures without compromising the skin. A 20-minute rest period between icing allows the skin to return to normal while deeper tissue temperature remains low.

Don't exercise within 30 minutes after icing. Reflex activity and motor functions are impaired which make you susceptible to injury. Avoid heating pads or hot tubs. Heat actually raises tissue temperatures, increasing circulation, which can cause more swelling and pain.

 Fiction
If your muscles are sore, you worked out too hard.

 Fact
If your muscles aren't sore, you didn't work out hard enough. Once the damage has occurred to the muscles, they rebuild stronger than before.

chapter 28

Get Enough Sleep

We build muscle when we rest and sleep, not when we're working out. Older people need more sleep and rest to recover than younger people. The older we are, the more rest we need. When working for a fat-to-muscle transition, middle age people need 8 1/2 to 9 hours of sleep per night.

This may sound like a lot of sleep to those of us who are used to getting no more than seven. A study published by Tufts University of Health and Nutrition Letter in 1989 explains why sleep is so important. Researchers discovered that, "people who slept an average of seven hours a night had significantly higher levels of cortisol in the afternoon than when they slept for nine hours a night." The effects of elevated cortisol levels from lack of sleep or stress may cause our bodies to start cannibalizing muscle, resulting in an increase of body fat accumulation around the belly.

Weight training creates a lot of cell-damaging free radicals in our bodies. Getting enough sleep will help us get rid of these toxins and improve our immune systems. Drs. Ingibjorg Jonsdottir and Pavel Hoffman from Sweden injected cancer cells into rats that exercised. They found that the animals improved their immune function – as measured by their ability to get rid of cancer cells – after eleven weeks of training. When training, your immune system will be your friend, but only if you get enough sleep.

PART 6

What We Should
Know About Body Fat

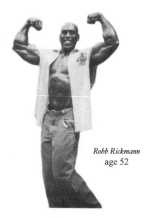

Robb Rickmann
age 52

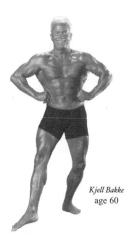

Kjell Bakke
age 60

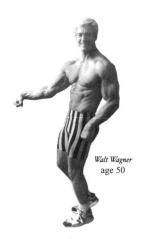

Walt Wagner
age 50

chapter 29

Optimal Body Fat

Men lose body fat more easily than women because testosterone levels in men are higher, thus helping men maintain more muscle mass. The hormone systems of women resist changes in the body composition as a protective mechanism that helps conserve energy during pregnancy. Most women find it difficult to maintain a body fat percentage lower than 12%, whereas it is not uncommon for athletic men to stay around 6%.

Extreme athletes like marathoners, wrestlers and competitive bodybuilders drop down below 4% or lower. The long term effects from going this low are unknown. Recent research proved that rats, which were put on special diets to considerably lower their body fat levels, lived twice as long as normal rats. I can tell you from experience that staying this low for extended periods is "pushing the envelope". You risk injuries, bruise easily, are cold even in moderate weather, don't recover from workouts as fast, are weaker and become mentally stressed more easily.

For males over 50 years old, the optimal body fat percentage is 20-28%. For women over 50 years old, the optimal range is 23-34%. These numbers are only approximations. It doesn't mean a male at 6% or a woman at 10% isn't healthy.

Body fat guidelines are useful as general guidelines; they are best used as subjective appraisal. Our ideal body fat percentage is where we look and feel best. Check the following body fat scale to see if you are athletic, optimal, or overfat. What body fat percentage would you like to be? Set a realistic goal for yourself.

Body Fat Range

	OPTIMAL FITNESS	
	Over 30 Yrs.	Over 50 Yrs.
Males	13-23%	20-28%
Females	17-30%	23-34%
	ATHLETIC	
Males	4-12%	5-19%
Females	10-19%	12-22%
	OVERFAT	
Males	over 23%	over 28%
Females	over 30%	over 34%

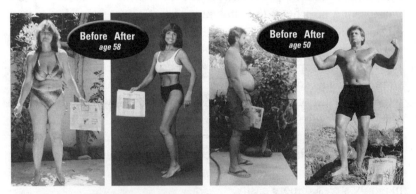

(From front cover) Joyce Linschoten and Dennis Strahl changed their physiques in less than four months following the **Muscle & Longevity** *philosophy, and they have kept the extra weight off.*

chapter 30 # Good Fat - Bad Fat

For the last 20 years, we've been told with almost religious certainty by everyone from the Surgeon General on down, that obesity is caused by the excessive consumption of fat, and that if we eat less fat we will lose weight and live longer.

Fat consumption in the U.S. has dropped from 40% to 30% in the last 20 years. Our supermarket shelves are full of "low fat" and "non-fat" foods. Why, then, has obesity jumped 30%? Why are we eating less fat and getting fatter? Put simply, the low fat diet has been a miserable failure.

The obesity epidemic started around the early 1980's. According to Katherine Flegal, an epidemiologist at the National Center for Health Statistics, the percentage of obese Americans stayed relatively constant through the 1960's and 1970's at 13% and then jumped 8 percentage points in the 1980's.

4"

1 lb. of body fat (simulation)

This steep rise has continued unabated to present time.

We do need fat in our diets to survive. Fat is vital to daily bodily functions: it cushions our joints, kidneys, liver and nerves. Body fat provides insulation against cold, keeps us alive when food is scarce and acts as a carrier for fat-soluble vitamins. Fat is needed to transport cholesterol build-up off the artery walls and bring it to the liver for processing. If we eat too much fat, however, our bodies store it as body fat. *Fat is fat – we either burn it or store it!* Each pound of body fat contains 3,500 calories. A person who is 20 pounds overfat has a 70,000 calorie surplus.

Unlike muscle, body fat doesn't burn any calories. Fat takes up more space than muscle. It's bulky and less dense. Each fat gram contains 9 calories as compared to 4 calories for each gram of protein or carbohydrate. Calories from fat are metabolized differently than calories from protein and carbohydrates. A pound of muscle is about 30% smaller than a pound of fat.

The more overfat we are, the less efficient we become at burning fat. That's why overfat people get tired much faster than fit people. Overfat people burn glucose, and our bodies don't store glucose like fat.

Fat-Free Food Can Make Us Fat

The government has spent over 300 million dollars in research projects trying to figure out why we keep getting fatter. The obvious explanation is what Kelly Brownell, a Yale psychologist, has called a "toxic food environment" of cheap over-processed food, large portions, pervasive food advertising and sedentary lifestyles.

Thank the wizardry of the food processors. "Fat-free" doesn't mean calorie free. *By replacing fat with sugar the average American eats 20% more calories today than 20 years ago.* Many regard "fat-free" as a green light to eat as much as they want.

If you eat five "reduced-fat" Oreos you are actually eating more calories than if you ate three regular Oreos. A "reduced fat" Oreo has only ten fewer calories than a regular Oreo (43 vs. 53), so five "reduced-fat" Oreos have 215 calories – 56 more than three regular Oreos (159). Eating more "low fat" food is as bad, or worse, than eating too much fat. This is why processed, high glycemic, calorie rich foods are the single biggest cause of obesity in America today.

Fat In Its Various Forms

Fats can be divided into four types: *monounsaturated, polyunsaturated, saturated,* and *trans fat.*

Monounsaturated fat, a good fat, is found in olives, almonds, pecans, cashews, peanuts, avocados and canola (rapeseed) oil. Monounsaturated fats are usually liquid at room temperature.

Avoid polyunsaturated fats touted as health foods, found in soy, cottonseed, corn and safflower oil. These oils are almost always rancid and most have a very high Omega-6 component.

Although the government's new dietary guidelines advise us to avoid it, saturated fat from animal sources is healthy when consumed in limited quantities. Saturated fats form a solid or semisolid fat at room temperature.

Recently, scientists have discovered trans fat to be very dangerous. Trans fat is formed during the hydrogenation process commonly used in the over processing of vegetable oils. Avoid trans fat found in hydrogenated food; it only clogs our arteries.

Cooking Oil & Salad Dressing

Many people don't realize salad dressings and cooking oils have extremely high fat contents. I've seen numerous people who are trying to lose body fat order a healthy salad and then dump 6 teaspoons of bleu cheese salad dressing on it, not realizing they're consuming nearly 50 grams of fat. Or they may cook a healthy serving of cod fish in the frying pan with 6 tablespoons of olive oil which adds 57 fat grams. This should be their total fat consumption for two days!

Steam food, or fry it in lemon juice. Use balsamic vinegar on your salads. Even low fat or non fat dressings have high sugar content. Don't eat corn oil or fish oil… it's processed. Eat corn and fish – food in its natural form – to get the essential fatty acids you need.

Eat Fat To Lose Body Fat

The *Muscle & Longevity* program utilizes a "good-fat" diet. If you're trying to lose body fat, limit your fat intake to no more than 15% of your total daily caloric intake. If you would like to see proof that this limited "good fat" program works, look at the before and after photos of people in this book. What better evidence is there?

Generally speaking, after you reach your desired body fat percentage, you can increase your fat consumption to around 20% from good sources without gaining body fat. No two people are the same; experiment using your body fat as a guide. If you start gaining body fat, reduce your fat intake.

When we supply our bodies with the optimal daily caloric intake from good fat, fat will be our ally in the battle to lose body fat and increase lean muscle. Fat is our first choice of fuel – not only the fat we eat, but stored body fat – *but only if we create a calorie deficit.*

On the other hand, if we restrict our fat intake too much, we not only deprive our bodies of a vital nutrient, we also force it to use carbs and protein for daily energy requirements, leaving little for growth.

Omega 3 fats (found in cold-water fish and flaxseed oil) naturally help our bodies burn fat. They do this by increasing the activity of carnitine in our bodies and by helping our cells (especially muscle cells) respond better to insulin to burn calories more effectively.

The Omega 3's found in flaxseed oil are so readily oxidized that they burn off nearly as fast as carbohydrates, greatly increasing the energy mechanisms in cells. These Omega 3's burn more quickly than other fats and raise our metabolism, providing energy to exercise longer. They are so energizing they may actually keep us awake at night if we take them before going to bed. Studies have led researchers to conclude Omega-3's may help prevent and even reverse obesity. They are often referred to as "the anti-obesity" fats.

When you are trying to lose body fat, it is paradoxical that you have to eat fat to lose fat. This is because as you begin to lose fat, Omega-3 fats are the first to go. This is ironic, considering that the most important fats are the ones most quickly burned off, but it's true. Not only will you lose body fat faster, you'll keep it off by supplementing Omega-3's. This is why we should take one teaspoon of flaxseed oil each day as we reduce body fat or eat one serving of cold-water fish each day. This is especially important if we are in ketosis, for helping the body deal with this steady body fat loss.

Consumed when we are young, Omega-3's also help prevent the development of an excessive number of fat cells. This helps prevent us from being overfat as we age.

❓ Fiction
The more body fat we have, the more body fat we burn.

❗ Fact
The more body fat we have, the less body fat we burn.

chapter 31 # Your Biology Isn't Your Destiny

Depending on genetic make-up, some people have more body fat and some have less. There are three distinctive body classifications based on physique, known as somatotypes. The three somatotype classifications are ectomorph, endomorph, and mesomorph.

An *ectomorph*, (Ted Danson), is a person whose lean and lanky physique is characterized by a slender build with long limbs, an angular profile, and prominent muscles or bones.

A *mesomorph*, (Sylvester Stallone), is a person whose physique is characterized by a well-proportioned, muscular body with broad shoulders, thick neck, deep chest and flat abdomen.

An *endomorph*, (Richard Simmons), is a person whose pear shaped physique is characterized by a soft, round physique with a large trunk and thighs, tapering extremities, an accumulation of fat throughout the body, short round limbs, a full face, a short neck, stockiness, and a tendency toward obesity.

People can have characteristics of more than one somatotype. A brief review of somatotypes reveals a numerical system assigned to fit each person. Every person is ranked from one to seven, based on his or her tendency to trait characteristics of each somatotype.

For example, a tall, thin, but muscular basketball player might be

Same weight, different somatotype

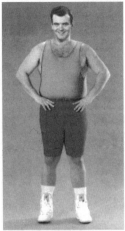 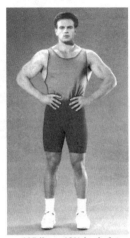

185 lbs. - 40% body fat   185 lbs. - 10% body fat

Body fat percentage, not weight, is the more accurate indicator of your physical health. For instance, both these men weigh the same, but the man on the left has 40% body fat, whereas the man on the right has 10% body fat.

considered a 5-4-1. (ectomorph, mesomorph, endomorph respectively). A muscular prize fighter might be considered a 1-7-1. What type of somatotype (body type) did you inherit?

Genetic shortcomings are easily applied to the somatotypes that frequent the gym. Skinny people complain because they don't put on muscle and overfat people complain because they can't seem to lose body fat.

I've seen many people totally change their somatotypes with exercise and diet, but it takes years, not months. Even with genetic shortcomings, we can usually prevent problems like obesity, high blood pressure, diabetes, heart disease, high cholesterol or cancer on the *Muscle & Longevity* program. Most people can overcome their genetic shortcomings for a long, healthy life.

I'm a good example. My mother, father and grandfathers all had a history of cardiovascular disease. Their cholesterol was very high, as with my brother and myself. I was on two kinds of cholesterol lowering drugs. My immune system was low. I used to get sick at least twice a year. After 90 days on the *Muscle and Longevity* program, I stopped taking the medications and haven't been sick for a single day. That was over five years ago!

There is no perfect exercise or diet for everyone. We're all different. You should customize your workouts and diet to achieve your individual goals.

chapter 32

Why Diets Don't Work

I t is important to realize that altered body composition and fitness goals are gained through fat loss
and muscle gain, not weight loss. Rapid weight loss
and undereating cause muscle tissue to be used for energy, which
decreases metabolism. Eating foods and supplements that fuel muscle
tissue will help you burn fat efficiently during exercise and at rest.

Calories are burned in muscle tissue. One pound of lean body
mass burns approximately 15-50 calories daily (depending on activity) and stores 450 calories of energy. Conversely, body fat is a store-
house for calories. One pound of fat burns approximately six calories
daily and stores 3,500 calories. Muscle tissue is more dense than fat
tissue because it is 70% water, while fat is about 20% water.

When you lose weight quickly (more than a few pounds a week),
most of the weight loss comes from water and muscle, not body fat.
When we stop dieting we gain the weight back with change – our
body's way of protecting us from the next famine. That's why conventional dieting is a vicious circle of weight loss and gain.

This is why typical calorie restriction (CR) diets don't work.
Neither do diets that eliminate entire food groups. Our bodies have
over 60 genes that help protect fat stores so we won't die from
starvation.

This Graph Shows Why Typical Diets Don't Work

REALITY **WEIGHT**

TYPICAL DIET BEGINS:

Starting calories 1,500 (500 calorie deficit)
Person must be in a caloric deficit to lose weight. ● **160 LBS**

Body must now learn to survive on 1,500 calories daily. Internal survival mechanisms are activated.

Body adapts by getting rid of the tissue that uses calories: muscle.

The body now has less muscle to feed, therefore it can survive on 1,500, rather than 2,000 calories daily. ● **145 LBS**

INITIAL RESULT
Early Plateau:

Body no longer loses weight because it is no longer in a caloric deficit. The body now receives and burns only 1,500 calories daily.

DIET ADJUSTMENT:

Person must drop to a new energy deficit to continue to lose weight (i.e., cut calories).

New maintenance:	1,500 calories.
New diet:	1,000 calories.
Deficit:	500 calories.

WEIGHT LOSS STARTS AGAIN:

Body must repeat muscle and fat loss until it is able to function on 1,000 calories as it did on 1,500 calories. ● **135 LBS**

WEIGHT LOSS STOPS AGAIN:

Now able to run on 1,000 calories, the body is closer to starvation and therefore activates additional energy saving tactics: endocrine system slows, more than 50 percent weight loss is derived from muscle tissue which causes lethargy. Decrease in energy leads to decrease in activity. Fewer calories are burned due to lack of activity and loss of muscle tissue.

FINAL PLATEAU:

At this point, there is nowhere else to go: calories cannot be futher decreased; a significant loss of fat burning tissue (muscle) has occured; slowing of the endocrine system; decreased energy. Weight loss is practically impossible and weight gain is inevitable because the hunger is uncontrollable.

TEMPORARY RESULT:

Gross weight loss:	25 pounds
Muscle loss:	15 pounds
Fat loss:	10 pounds

CONCLUDING STATISTICS:

Weight:	135 pounds
Body fat:	30 percent
Hunger level:	Insatiable

Current caloric intake to maintain new body composition: 1,000 calories daily. Basically, the person is a smaller version of his/her former self, has a lowered metobolic rate and is incurably hungry.

THE INEVITABLE ROAD BACK

WEIGHT GAIN:
Body Fat

The body had adapted to 1,000 calories to maintain current body composition and activity. As a result, any additional calories are unnecessary and will be stored as fat.

Continual hunger and new cravings will eventually result in an increase in caloric intake. Body fat will increase to the original set point, or higher, in order to prepare the body for another bout with starvation (i.e., dieting).

THE END RESULT:

1 Year Later:
165 lbs.
38% body fat
Caloric intake necessary to maintain current body composition: 1,500 calories daily. Dieter shops for another plan or magic formula.

When we severely cut calories or entire food groups, our metabolisms slow down to preserve fat supplies. Our fat cells begin to produce a hormone called leptin that helps us store more fat. Our brains release neuropeptide-Y, which causes intense food cravings, and we start burning muscle instead of fat.

There are a lot of ways to lose weight. We can cut carbs, cut fat, or reduce calories – they will all work, at least temporarily. Losing weight doesn't make us healthy, our body fat-to-muscle ratio does.

The 90 day *Muscle & Longevity* program works because we only reduce calories from high glycemic carbs, eat balanced meals often, supplement and exercise properly to build muscle while burning fat.

Original Statistics:	Weight:	160 pounds
	Body fat:	32%
	Hunger level:	Satisfied

Current caloric intake to maintain body composition: 2,000 calories daily.
Goal Weight: 125 pounds

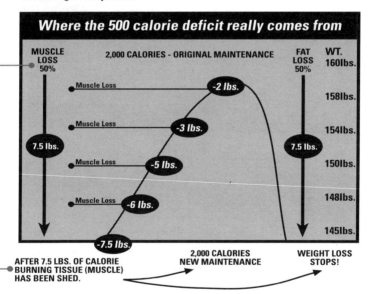

Fiction
We should severely cut calories to lose weight.

Fact
We should eat small balanced meals every few hours to lose body fat.

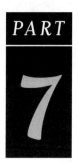

PART

7

Six Steps To Fitness

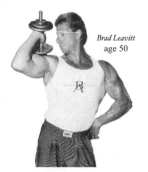

Brad Leavitt
age 50

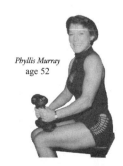

Phyllis Murray
age 52

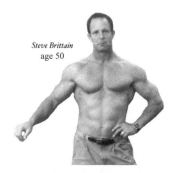

Steve Brittain
age 50

chapter 33

Step 1: Plan Your Fitness Goal

Most people in the gym aren't following a fitness program with specific goals. As a result, they don't make the gains they could. Humans are goal oriented. On the *Muscle & Longevity* program body fat percentage is used as a foundation in determining your fitness goals. These include your current body fat-to-muscle ratio, ideal body fat goal and how much weight you need to lose to reach your body fat goal.

Measuring your body fat percentage

To determine your fitness goals, the first thing you need to know is your current body fat percentage. Your body fat percentage, not your weight, defines how fit you are. You need to know what percentage of your weight is fat vs. lean muscle mass. Your local trainer can measure your body fat percentage or you can buy body fat calipers or body fat scales and do it yourself (See Suppliers Directory).

Although the calipers are extremely accurate, the body fat scales are the the easiest to use. Just stand on them in your bare feet and they give you a readout of your weight and body fat. Take this reading every morning before eating or drinking anything for a more accurate reading. Keep a daily progress record. This will provide you an excellent indicator of your progress.

Body Fat Calipers

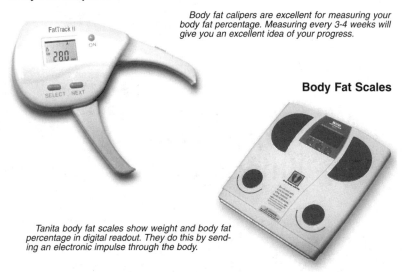

Body fat calipers are excellent for measuring your body fat percentage. Measuring every 3-4 weeks will give you an excellent idea of your progress.

Body Fat Scales

Tanita body fat scales show weight and body fat percentage in digital readout. They do this by sending an electronic impulse through the body.

How do we know how much weight to lose?

Once you know your body fat percentage, it's easy to figure out how much weight you need to lose. Let's say you decide you want to reach 15% body fat and you weigh 185 pounds with 30% body fat.

First, multiply your current weight by your body fat percentage (185 x .30 = 55 lb.) to determine your pounds of body fat. Then, subtract your body fat weight from your current total weight to give you your net body weight (185 – 55 = 130). Next, divide your net body weight by .85 which is the same as saying that you shouldn't weigh more than your muscle plus 15% fat (130 divided by .85 = 153).

In the example, you would need to lose 32 pounds of fat, (185 – 153 = 32 pounds) to achieve 15% body fat. This formula works for any size or somatotype. Enter this information onto your Tracking Record on the page 133.

Formula for figuring how much weight to lose	
(185 lb person as example)	
185 X .30 = 55 lbs.	Body Fat
185 – 56 = 130 lbs.	Muscle
130 ÷ .85 = 153 lbs.	Ideal Weight Goal
185 – 153 = 32 lbs.	Weight to lose to reach 15% body fat

Making Time For Fitness

Once you figure out how much fat you have to lose to get fit, you need to set up a regular workout schedule. One of the most popular excuses for not working out is *not having enough time.*

Many of us often spend time on things that really aren't top priorities. If you frequently use time as an excuse for missing workouts, here are some ways to see if that excuse is valid. Being totally objective, list the top eight items that are most important to you (1 = most important).

LIST 1. *Most important things in my life:*

1. _____
2. _____
3. _____
4. _____
5. _____
6. _____
7. _____
8. _____

Now, list the top eight ways you currently spend your time (1 = the activity you spend the most time on).

LIST 2. *How I spend my time:*

1. _____
2. _____
3. _____
5. _____
6. _____
7. _____
8. _____

Examine list #2 and see if you can cut ten or twenty minutes off things like talking on the phone, watching television, eating at restaurants, etc. List each activity and time wasted below.

LIST 3. *Time I waste daily:*

	Activity	Time wasted daily (minutes)
1.	_____	_____
2.	_____	_____
3.	_____	_____
4.	_____	_____
5.	_____	_____
6.	_____	_____
7.	_____	_____
8.	_____	_____

Compare list 1 with list 2. How much time do you actually devote to what you really consider important? Do you waste time on activities that aren't that important to you? If your two lists don't match, it's time to get your priorities in line.

Now look at list 3. It shows how much time you waste and that planing your time more wisely can free up time for exercise. It's simply a matter of motivation. Your health is the most valuable possession you have.

? **Fiction**
Cholesterol is the best indicator of physical health.

! **Fact**
Body fat is the best indicator of physical health.

Your Tracking Record

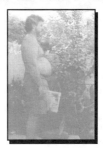 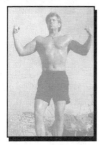

before body fat %_____

Date: _____

Starting body fat % _____

Goal body fat % _____

Body Measurements Before:

Biceps _____

Waist _____   Thighs _____

Chest _____   Hips (women) _____

Follow this formula to determine how much weight you need to lose.

185 lbs.	X	.30	=	55 lbs.
weight		body fat %		lbs. body fat

185 lbs.	−	55 lbs.	=	153 lbs.
weight		body fat		lbs. muscle

130 lbs.	÷	130 ÷ .85	=	153 lbs.
lbs. muscle		lbs. divided by 100 – desired body fat percentage (100 – 15 = .85)		body weight at desired body fat percentage (15%)

Weight I need to lose to achieve desired body fat percentage.

 pounds to lose   goal body weight pounds

100%   Daily Maintenance Caloric requirement _____calories

75%   Daily Maintenance Caloric requirement *(to reduce body fat)*_____calories

chapter 34

Step 2: Reduce Caloric Intake

Basil Metabolic Rate (BMR) is the number of calories your body uses to simply exist, as if you were in a coma. For instance, an average athletic 5'2", 130 pound woman's BMR would be around 1,000. Adding daily activities, workouts and digestion to the scenario would bring her total daily maintenance caloric requirements (DMC) to around 1,600.

Most people require about ten calories per pound of body weight per day just to stay alive. So an inactive 200 pound man requires a minimum of 2,000 calories. For most people who are active at work and home, the ideal daily intake for weight maintenance is 12-15 calories per pound.

If your goal is to burn excess body fat, *reduce your daily caloric intake to about 75% of your DMC requirement.* To determine your DMC, check the chart on page 138-139. Although this chart is accurate for most people, athletic people with high metabolic rates or sedentary people with lower metabolic rates need to adjust their intake. For instance, I know from the chart my daily DMC is 2,169, so I adjust my daily caloric intake to 2,300 calories because I'm muscular and athletic, with a higher metabolic rate than normal.

Most people will lose about a pound a week. For instance, if your DMC requirement is 2,000 per day, and you reduce it to 1,500 by cutting 500 calories per day, you'll be burning an extra 3,500 calories per week (500 x 7=3,500). There are 3,500 calories in one pound. The calories have to come from somewhere; it's a medical certainty.

During the first month of the 90 day program, the objective is to achieve ketosis. Ketosis burns body fat in a safe and effective way, maintaining a balanced 40% low glycemic carbs, 45% protein, 15% *good* fat ratio at each meal. (Oatmeal at breakfast is the exception as it is considered mid-high glycemic.)

Unlike most diets, you probably won't start losing weight until the end of the third week. This is because with most diets the weight loss is mostly water and muscle – with the *Muscle & Longevity* diet, it's mostly body fat.

The first two or three weeks, reduce your caloric intake about 10%. The calorie reductions should come from each balanced meal. When cutting calories, first cut food containing dietary fats, saturated fats, cholesterol and sugar. Reduce this type of calories because they are the major fat-causing culprits in any diet. Complex carbs should only be reduced the last month at a minimum because they help to maintain blood-sugar levels and supply a steady flow of energy. About one month into the program you want to be at 75% of your DMC.

If you reach a "sticking point" and stop losing body fat, slightly reduce caloric intake, but do it in very small steps by reducing the food types discussed above. You can also increase the time of your cardio workouts from 20 to 30 minutes to help get yourself through the sticking point. Just make sure you stay in your aerobic heart rate zone.

You might need to vary your caloric intake every few weeks. This is because your body might adjust to your new sub-maintenance caloric intake by lowering your BMR. Eating small meals with protein every few hours will usually prevent this, by "tricking" your body into thinking you are eating more than you are.

Proteins should never be reduced when cutting calories. Amino acids are the last source of energy the body has and their primary function is to repair and rebuild muscle tissues. *The body ends up burning more calories digesting and processing protein than it derives from the protein consumed.*

It is easier to monitor your caloric intake by eliminating "hidden" calories such as those found in sauces, salad dressings, cooking oils and processed foods. You can count daily calories using the following figures.

1 gram of fat = 9 calories	**1 gram of carbs** = 4 calories
1 gram of protein = 4 calories	**1 gram of alcohol** = 7 calories

Rather than counting calories, it is easier just to follow the sample 2,300 CR diet on page 140. Adjust portion sizes to meet your caloric requirements. You'll know if your portions are too big if you're not losing body fat. If you don't like the food or get tired of eating the same thing, you can substitute from the substitute food list at end of the chapter.

As you increase your ratio of muscle to body fat, your metabolism will increase. In time, you may end up actually weighing the same as when you started the program, but you'll be more fit because muscle weighs more than fat.

As an example, I weigh 185 pounds now – the same as when I started the *Muscle & Longevity* program five years ago – but my body fat has gone from 25% to 8%.

This means I've replaced 30 pounds of fat with 30 pounds of muscle. That's 6 pounds of muscle gain per year, which is not uncommon on the *Muscle & Longevity* program. Most people lose their extra body fat in the first 90 days and then make steady muscle gains until they reach their genetic potential, which usually takes about 6 years.

A Healthy Breakfast For Fat-To-Muscle Transition

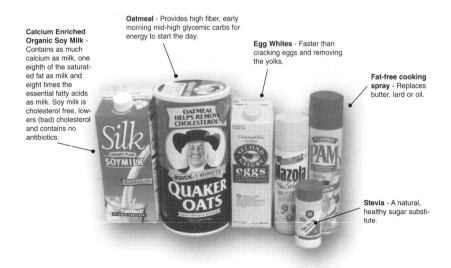

Calcium Enriched Organic Soy Milk - Contains as much calcium as milk, one eighth of the saturated fat as milk and eight times the essential fatty acids as milk. Soy milk is cholesterol free, lowers (bad) cholesterol and contains no antibiotics.

Oatmeal - Provides high fiber, early morning mid-high glycemic carbs for energy to start the day.

Egg Whites - Faster than cracking eggs and removing the yolks.

Fat-free cooking spray - Replaces butter, lard or oil.

Stevia - A natural, healthy sugar substitute.

The Largest Meal Of the Day - *In the morning after your aerobic exercise, your body needs a big breakfast to keep from regressing to a starvation mode. Although these foods are processed, they are not over-processed. I add free-range chicken, fish or turkey and veggies to the egg whites for a fast, nutritional omelette.*

Calorie Intake Chart For Women

Weight In Pounds

Height in Inches

Weight	%	57	58	59	60	61	62	63	64	65	66	67	68	69	70	71	72
80	125%	2045	2085	2185	2170	2210	2245	2275	2312	2345	2370	2400	2420	2455	2480	2505	2532
	100%	1315	1325	1345	1355	1372	1385	1398	1405	1415	1430	1440	1450	1460	1470	1475	1483
	70%	920	930	940	950	960	965	975	987	990	1001	1010	1015	1020	1030	1035	1040
90	125%	1682	1705	1725	1745	1760	1780	1795	1815	1830	1845	1860	1875	1885	1900	1910	1925
	100%	1345	1365	1375	1395	1410	1425	1440	1450	1465	1478	1490	1495	1510	1520	1530	1540
	70%	940	955	967	975	990	995	1010	1017	1025	1035	1040	1050	1055	1065	1073	1075
100	125%	1722	1747	1770	1792	1810	1830	1853	1870	1885	1905	1920	1933	1950	1965	1975	1995
	100%	1375	1395	1415	1435	1450	1467	1485	1498	1510	1525	1535	1550	1560	1570	1580	1590
	70%	965	975	992	1005	1015	1027	1040	1045	1055	1065	1073	1085	1090	1102	1110	1117
110	125%	1760	1785	1815	1835	1863	1885	1905	1925	1945	1960	1980	1995	2015	2030	2045	2060
	100%	1410	1433	1452	1473	1490	1510	1525	1540	1555	1570	1585	1595	1612	1625	1633	1645
	70%	990	1000	1017	1030	1045	1055	1065	1075	1090	1095	1110	1115	1125	1140	1145	1150
120	125%	1800	1835	1860	1887	1912	1935	1960	1980	2002	2022	2043	2060	2075	2095	2112	2124
	100%	1440	1465	1490	1510	1525	1545	1565	1580	1602	1615	1635	1645	1660	1675	1685	1703
	70%	1010	1027	1045	1057	1070	1085	1095	1110	1122	1130	1145	1150	1165	1175	1180	1187
130	125%	1845	1875	1905	1930	1960	1987	2012	2035	2055	2080	2103	2123	2140	2160	2175	2195
	100%	1475	1500	1525	1545	1565	1585	1610	1625	1645	1665	1683	1695	1710	1725	1740	1755
	70%	1030	1050	1065	1080	1095	1115	1128	1140	1150	1165	1175	1190	1195	1210	1215	1225
140	125%	1885	1915	1950	1980	2010	2035	2065	2090	2115	2135	2163	2183	2205	2225	2245	2263
	100%	1505	1535	1560	1585	1605	1630	1650	1675	1690	1713	1725	1743	1765	1775	1795	1805
	70%	1055	1075	1090	1110	1127	1140	1155	1173	1185	1200	1212	1225	1235	1240	1259	1265
150	125%	1925	1960	1995	2030	2060	2085	2115	2147	2170	2195	2222	2245	2265	2285	2305	2330
	100%	1540	1565	1598	1620	1645	1670	1695	1715	1735	1755	1775	1793	1815	1833	1845	1865
	70%	1080	1095	1115	1137	1150	1170	1185	1200	1215	1233	1245	1255	1270	1280	1295	1305
160	125%	1965	2005	2040	2075	2110	2145	2173	2203	2230	2253	2280	2305	2330	2350	2375	2396
	100%	1573	1600	1630	1660	1685	1715	1735	1763	1785	1805	1823	1845	1865	1885	1895	1915
	70%	1100	1120	1145	1160	1183	1195	1217	1235	1245	1265	1275	1290	1305	1315	1330	1340
170	125%	2005	2047	2085	2120	2155	2190	2225	2257	2288	2315	2340	2395	2395	2415	2443	2460
	100%	1605	1635	1665	1695	1725	1755	1780	1805	1830	1850	1875	1895	1915	1930	1955	1973
	70%	1120	1143	1165	1185	1210	1225	1248	1265	1282	1295	1315	1325	1342	1355	1365	1375
180	125%	2045	2090	2130	2170	2210	2245	2275	2315	2345	2375	2400	2430	2455	2485	2505	2535
	100%	1635	1675	1705	2638	1768	1795	1825	1845	1875	1895	1920	1945	1968	1990	2000	2025
	70%	1150	1170	1195	1215	1235	1255	1278	1295	1315	1325	1340	1365	1378	1395	1405	1415
190	125%	2085	2130	2170	2210	2250	2285	2320	2355	2385	2415	2440	2470	2500	2525	2545	2575
	100%	1665	1705	1738	1770	1795	1825	1855	1885	1910	1935	1955	1980	1995	2020	2040	2055
	70%	1165	1190	1217	1240	1260	1280	1295	1315	1335	1350	1365	1385	1395	1415	1425	1445
200	125%	2125	2170	2210	2250	2290	2325	2360	2395	2425	2450	2480	2510	2335	2565	2585	2615
	100%	1700	1735	1765	1800	1830	1860	1890	1915	1940	1965	1990	2010	2030	2050	2070	2090
	70%	1190	1217	1240	1265	1285	1305	1320	1345	1360	1375	1390	1405	1420	1435	1450	1465
210	125%	2165	2210	2250	2290	2325	2365	2435	2465	2495	2520	2550	2575	2600	2625	2655	
	100%	1730	1765	1800	1830	1860	1895	1920	1945	1975	1995	2020	2040	2060	2080	2100	2125
	70%	1215	1235	1260	1285	1303	1329	1345	1365	1385	1395	1415	1430	1445	1460	1475	1490
220	125%	2205	2245	2290	2330	2365	2405	2440	2475	2505	2530	2560	2590	2615	2640	2665	2695
	100%	1765	1795	1830	1865	1895	1925	1955	1975	2005	2025	2050	2070	2095	2115	2135	2155
	70%	1235	1260	1285	1310	1325	1350	1365	1390	1405	1425	1440	1450	1465	1485	1490	1510
230	125%	2245	2285	2330	2370	2405	2445	2475	2515	2545	2575	2600	2630	2655	2685	2705	2735
	100%	1798	1835	1865	1898	1930	1955	1985	2010	2035	2055	2080	2100	2125	2150	2175	2185
	70%	1265	1285	1310	1330	1350	1370	1395	1410	1425	1445	1465	1478	1495	1500	1515	1535
240	125%	2285	2330	2370	2410	2450	2485	2520	2555	2585	2615	2640	2670	2695	2725	2745	2775
	100%	1825	1865	1898	1930	1960	1990	2015	2045	2065	2095	2115	2140	2155	2175	2210	2215
	70%	1285	1310	1335	1350	1375	1395	1415	1435	1450	1465	1485	1500	1515	1525	1540	1550
250	125%	2325	2370	2410	2450	2485	2525	2560	2595	2625	2655	2680	2710	2735	2765	2785	2815
	100%	1860	1895	1930	1960	1990	2020	2045	2075	2095	2125	2150	2170	2190	2210	2240	2250
	70%	1305	1335	1355	1360	1395	1420	1435	1460	1475	1490	1505	1520	1535	1550	1565	1580

Calorie Intake Chart For Men

Weight In
Pounds

H e i g h t   i n   I n c h e s

		60	61	62	63	64	65	66	67	68	69	70	71	72	73	74	75
110	125%	1935	1970	2005	2040	2065	2095	2125	2155	2180	2205	2230	2255	2275	2290	2320	2340
	100%	1550	1575	1605	1635	1650	1675	1700	1725	1745	1760	1785	1805	1820	1840	1855	1875
	70%	1080	1105	1120	1140	1155	1175	1190	1205	1215	1235	1250	1265	1275	1280	1295	1310
120	125%	2005	2050	2075	2110	2135	2165	2190	2225	2250	2275	2295	2325	2350	2365	2390	2410
	100%	1605	1630	1660	1680	1715	1735	1755	1775	1795	1825	1840	1860	1875	1890	1910	1925
	70%	1120	1140	1165	1180	1190	1210	1230	1245	1260	1275	1285	1300	1315	1325	1335	1350
130	125%	2075	2110	2145	2175	2210	2235	2265	2290	2320	2345	2365	2390	2415	2440	2455	2475
	100%	1660	1685	1715	1745	1760	1785	1810	1835	1855	1880	1895	1915	1930	1950	1965	1985
	70%	1165	1185	1200	1215	1235	1250	1265	1285	1285	1315	1330	1340	1350	1365	1360	1385
140	125%	2145	2175	2210	2245	2275	2305	2335	2360	2385	2410	2435	2465	2485	2505	2525	2545
	100%	1715	1745	1770	1795	1825	1845	1865	1890	1910	1935	1950	1970	1985	2005	2025	2040
	70%	1200	1220	1240	1255	1275	1295	1305	1230	1335	1355	1365	1375	1395	1400	1415	1430
150	125%	2215	2250	2285	2315	2345	2375	2400	2430	2450	2480	2510	2530	2550	2575	2595	2620
	100%	1770	1795	1825	1855	1870	1895	1920	1945	1965	1985	2005	2025	2040	2060	2075	2090
	70%	1240	1255	1275	1290	1315	1330	1340	1365	1370	1390	1405	1415	1430	1440	1455	1465
160	125%	2280	2320	2355	2385	2420	2455	2485	2515	2540	2570	2595	2620	2645	2665	2690	2710
	100%	1830	1850	1885	1915	1935	1960	1985	2015	2035	2055	2070	2090	2120	2130	2150	2170
	70%	1275	1295	1315	1335	1355	1375	1390	1410	1425	1440	1455	1470	1485	1495	1505	1515
170	125%	2355	2395	2430	2465	2495	2535	2560	2595	2625	2650	2685	2710	2740	2765	2785	2810
	100%	1885	1915	1945	1970	2000	2025	2050	2075	2100	2125	2150	2170	2190	2210	2230	2245
	70%	1315	1340	1365	1385	1405	1420	1440	1455	1470	1490	1500	1515	1530	1545	1560	1570
180	125%	2420	2460	2500	2545	2575	2615	2650	2685	2710	2745	2775	2805	2830	2855	2880	2900
	100%	1940	1970	2000	2035	2060	2095	2220	2145	2170	2195	2220	2245	2260	2285	2305	2325
	70%	1360	1375	1400	1425	1445	1465	1480	1500	1520	1535	1550	1570	1585	1595	1615	1530
190	125%	2450	2530	2580	2620	2650	2695	2730	2765	2795	2830	2865	2895	2920	2950	2975	3000
	100%	1995	2025	2065	2095	2125	2155	2185	2210	2240	2265	2285	2315	2340	2360	2380	2400
	70%	1395	1420	1445	1460	1490	1510	1530	1550	1565	1585	1605	1610	1640	1655	1660	1685
200	125%	2560	2605	2650	2695	2735	2775	2810	2850	2885	2920	2950	2980	3010	3045	3070	3090
	100%	2050	2085	2120	2155	2190	2220	2250	2275	2305	2335	2360	2385	2410	2435	2460	2475
	70%	1432	1460	1485	1510	1530	1555	1575	1595	1615	1635	1650	1670	1685	1705	1715	1735

Determine your daily maintenance caloric requirements using these charts (women or men respectively) Using you weight and height, locate your 100% DMC. Then multiply times .75 to determine how many calories you should be eating on the **Muscle & Longevity** *90 day fat to muscle program.*

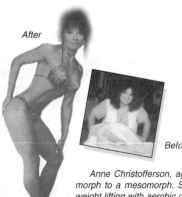

After

Before

Anne Christofferson, age 43, changed her somatotype from an endomorph to a mesomorph. She used the **Muscle & Longevity** *program of weight lifting with aerobic cross training, a low-glycemic, calorie restriction, smart fat diet and supplements.*

My Sample 2,300 Calorie Diet

Before morning cardio, drink 8 oz. of water. Do 20 minute aerobic exercise before breakfast.
Take supplements with breakfast

8:30 a.m.	Breakfast	1/2 grapefruit, 1 cup oatmeal with calcium & vitamin enriched non-GMO soy milk, sweeten with Stevia, 4 egg whites or egg beaters in a veggie omelet with broccoli, mushrooms, onions, & sprouts. Cook in non-fat cooking spray. coffee or tea, 8 oz. water.
10:30	snack	Protein supplement, green tea.
12:00	Lunch	4 oz. (the size of your fist), free range poultry or fish, Veggie salad with balsamic vinegar, 1 cup rice, 8 oz.water.
2:00	snack	1 can 2.7 oz. pop top solid white tuna in water, or protein supplement, 8 oz. water, green tea.
3:00	snack	1/2 apple, raw carrots, cauliflower or broccoli, 8 oz. water.
4:15	snack	1 can 2.7 oz. pop top solid white tuna in water, 5 grams creatine with 8 oz. water 45 minutes prior to weight lifting.
5:00	(training days only)	Weight training, 24 oz. water.
6:15	snack	Protein supplement, 8 oz. water.
7:00	Dinner	5 oz. lean wild, free range meat (bison, poultry or white ocean fish) small yam. Steamed vegetables (broccoli, brussel sprouts, asparagus, green beans, spinach), 8 oz. water, green tea.
8:00	snack	One serving raw vegetables, 4 oz. Orange Roughy or 1 tsp. organic flaxseed oil mixed with protein supplement, 8 oz. water.
9:00	snack	All the raw veggies I want, green tea.

Food Substitutes

If you don't like the food on the sample diet, you can exchange items listed below. This is necessary because if you don't like a certain food, you're less likely to stick to the diet. Plus, eating the same food gets boring. You can use this list to give yourself more choices.

Vegetables
Contain 25 calories and 5 grams of carbs. One serving equals:

1/2 cup	Cooked vegetables (broccoli, zucchini, cabbage, mushrooms, asparagus, cauliflower, green beans, brussels sprouts)
1-cup	Raw vegetables or salad greens
1/2 cup	Vegetable juice

Very Lean Protein (Steamed, broiled, or grilled with no added oil)
Choices have 35 calories and 1 gram of fat per serving. One serving equals:

1 ounce	Bison
1 ounce	Free-range turkey or chicken breast, skin removed
1 ounce	Fish filet (Orange Roughy, flounder, sole, halibut cod, etc.)
1 ounce	Canned tuna in water
1 ounce	Emu, ostrich, rabbit
1 ounce	Shellfish (clams, lobster, scallop, shrimp)
2 each	Egg whites
1/4 cup	Egg substitute
1/2 cup	Beans-cooked (black beans, kidney, chick peas or lentils)

Breads and starches
Each serving contains 15 grams of carbs and 80 calories

5 slices	Whole wheat melba toast
1 ounce	1/4 bagel (pumpernickel, whole wheat or white)
1/2 cup	Cooked cereal (oatmeal, cream of wheat, wheatina)
1/3 cup	Barley
1/3 cup	Rice-cooked, white, brown or wild
2 large	Round rice cakes, any flavor
1/2 cup	Corn, sweet potato, or yam
3 cups	Popcorn, hot air popped or microwave (80% light)

Fruits
Each serving provides 15 grams of carbs and 60 calories

1 cup	Fresh berries (strawberries, blueberries, raspberries)
1 medium	Apple, pear, nectarine
1/2 large	Grapefruit
1 small	Banana
1 cup	Fresh melon-cubes (honeydew or cantaloupe)
Small cluster	(15 each) grapes
1	Kiwi
1	Fresh peach

Fats
Each serving contains 5 grams of fat and 45 calories

1 teaspoon	Reduced fat peanut butter
6 whole	Walnuts, peanuts, almonds, mixed nuts or cashews
1 1/2 Tbls.	Trail mix
6 ounces	Tofu
1/8th	Avocado
8 large	Black olives
10 large	Green olives

Common Food Contents

Below are some common food items and their nutritional contents. For a complete book of most foods, read *Nutrition Almanac* by Lavon J. Dunne. (Data Source Nutritional Almanac, USA FDA, and *The T-Factor Diet* by Martin Kathahn, Ph. D.)

Food	Measure Weight	Calories	Protein grams	Fat grams
Meats				
Bison filet mignon	4 oz.	110	25	.5
Beef filet mignon	4 oz.	22	21	11.2
Ground bison	4 oz.	173	23	3
Ground beef (regular)	4 oz.	35	18.8	30
Pork chops	4 oz.	286	16	24
Spareribs	4 oz.	201	14	16.5
Liver	4 oz.	154	24	5
Bacon	4 oz.	631	10	65
Ham	4 oz.	207	20	22
Poultry				
Turkey (light	4 oz.	71.5	10	.8
Turkey (dark)	4 oz.	60	7	.87
Chicken (light)	4 oz.	54	6	.2
Chicken (dark)	4 oz.	95	7	2.25

Food	Measure Weight	Calories	Protein. grams	Fat grams
Luncheon & Sausage				
Bologna, beef	1 oz.	89	3.31	
Frankfurter, beef	1 oz.	145	5.08	
Seafood				
Salmon	3 oz.	121	16.9	5.39
Snapper	3 oz.	85	17.4	1.14
Halibut	3 oz.	93	17.7	1.95
Cod	3 oz.	70	15	.57
Orange Roughy	3 oz.	70	16	1
Crab	3 oz.	70	15	.51
Dairy & Eggs				
Whole Milk	1C	150	8.03	11.3
Low fat 2%	1C	121	8.12	4.68
Skim	1C	86	8.35	.44
Half & Half	1C	315	7.16	27.8
Whipping Cream (heavy)	1C	821	4.88	88
Cheddar Cheese	1 oz.	114	7.06	9.4
Sour Cream	1C	493	7.27	48.2
Vegetables				
Yams	1C	210	4.8	.4
Sweet Potato	1 (130 grm.)	136	2	.38
Peas, green	1C	118	7.9	.58
Kidney Beans	1C	218	14.4	.9
Carrots	1C	48	1	.2
Asparagus	1C	30	4.1	.3
Salad Dressing				
Bleu cheese	1T	77	.7	8
Italian	1T	68.7	.1	7.1
Thousand Island	1T	58.9	.1	5.6
Vinegar	1T	20	.9	0
Nuts				
Peanuts	1C	838	37.7	70.1
Peanut Butter	1T	86	3.9	8.1
Fruit & Fruit Juices				
Orange	1	62	1.23	.16
Grapes, slip skin	1C	58	.58	.32
Grape Juice	1C	155	1.4	.19
Apple	1	81	.27	.49
Banana	1	105	1.18	.55

Food	Measure Weight	Calories	Protein. grams	Fat grams
Frozen Desserts, Milk				
Ice Cream	1C	269	4.8	14.3
Ice Cream (rich)	1C	349	4.1	23.6
Cereals				
Corn Flakes, Kellogg's	1 1/4 C	110	2.3	.1
Oatmeal	1C	145	6	2.1
Shredded Wheat	1 lg.	83	2.6	.3
Bakery & Grains *(Most are high glycemic)*				
Crackers, soda	1	12.5	.26	7
Muffins, bran	1	104	3.1	3.9
Pancakes, buckwheat 4"	54	1.8	6.4	2.15
Pancakes, whole wheat 4"	74	3.	8.8	3 .2
Bagels	1	296	11	2.6
Rolls, dinner	1	113	3.1	2.2
White Bread 1 slice	62	2	11.6	.79
Whole Wheat 1 slice	56	2.4	11	.7
Pizza, cheese 14"	153	7.8	18.4	5 .4

Fiction
Skip breakfasts and eat only salads to lose weight and get fit.

Fact
Reduce caloric intake to 75% of your DMC requirements to achieve ketosis. Consume 1.5 grams of protein for each pound of body weight daily.

chapter 35

Step 3: Weight Training For A Fat-To-Muscle Transition

When targeting any muscle with a compound or multiple joint exercise, you train other muscles indirectly. For example, when you train your chest with dumbbell presses, you also work your triceps and deltoids indirectly. Your triceps get hit nearly as hard as your chest and your deltoids pick up the slack. This provides optimal direct/indirect workout relationships to achieve fat loss and muscle gain. Exercise large muscle groups first. As an example, work back first (a large muscle group), then work biceps (a smaller muscle group).

Rest a few minutes between each set (except abs, which you rest one minute between sets). Some people log their weight used in order to keep track of gains. Variety is important to maximize gains. Try to use a different exercise each week when working the same body part. For example, if you did bench press, pec deck and seated machine presses the last chest day, do incline, decline and flat bench with dumbbells the next chest day. *Changing routines increases gains.*

Breathing

Breathing is subtle, but very important when weight lifting. Although breathing is normally involuntary, you can control it. You can speed it up, slow it down, make it long and diaphragmatic, or make it short and thoracic. Controlled breathing requires immediate concentration. You can't be worrying about the future. You must be focused on the here-and-now.

Controlled breathing affects your entire psychological make-up, your hormones, your central nervous system, your autonomic nervous system, and even your heart rate. It helps predict and override situations that require immediate physical responses.

For instance, before curling dumbbells, your central nervous system sends a message to your brain to get ready for the activity. Just by anticipating a lift, your heart rate can jump as much as 100%. Before you lift, take a long breath deep from your diaphragm. As you lift, blow the air out. This tightens your muscles and sharpens concentration. As you let the weight down, slowly take another deep breath, preparing for the next repetition.

Time & Retention Weight Lifting

Over the years, normal weight lifting routines can lead to injuries. *These routines, which utilize full range of motion repetitions, nearly always lead to tendonitis, especially in older people.* This is due to the chronic impingement caused by many of the unnatural movements of many exercises using heavy weight.

In young people, these injuries usually show up about ten years later. In older folks, injuries show up in as little as three years. This is because older folks have more scar tissue in their tendons.

The way to help avoid these injuries is to avoid extremely heavy weight and minimize full range of motion movements. Unless you are a competitive weight lifter, there is no need to work with the maximum amount of weight you can lift. Instead of building up tendons and joints, you will only tear them up. Using heavy weight on unnatural movements like straight bar bench presses, over-head presses, French curls and deep squats will nearly always cause joint and/or tendon injuries.

The unique *Time & Retention* method of weight lifting helps prevent degeneration of tendons, ligaments and joints. Instead of doing many sets of full range of motion exercises with heavy weight, you start by warming up with 25-35 repetitions (reps) using light weight at the beginning of each exercise and stretch between sets. This warms up your muscles but reduces torque on the tendons and joints. Stretches should be held at least 15 seconds.

After you warm up, you're ready for the work set. Using your work weight (weight you can hold in the weakest part of the movement for 25-35 seconds), do a few full range reps, then move the weight to the weakest point of the movement.

Hold the weight in this position to total failure. *Total failure is until you can't possibly hold the weight another second. Don't quit when it starts to burn!* This sensation should be about halfway through the 25-35 seconds. If you can't reach 25-35 seconds, lighten the weight. If it is too easy, add weight. *Because most of the muscle hytrophy is achieved on the last 15 degrees of the negative movement, holding the weight in this position provides optimal stress for maximum gains.* Your heart rate will get up into your aerobic zone fast, because you're not resting at the top or bottom of the movement.

Train Smart, Train Safe

Seventy-five percent of all weight lifting injuries are shoulder and rotator cuff problems caused from doing straight bar bench presses. It is much safer to use dumbbells, rather than a straight bar for flat, incline and decline bench work because they place less stress on your

Time & Retention - hold the weight in the weakest part of the movement until failure. You will make gains fast and reduce chances for injury.

rotator. Don't clasp your hands behind your neck when doing sit-ups, cross them on your chest. Do seated cable lat pull-downs to your chest, not behind your neck.

Eliminate any movement which causes you discomfort. There are many other safe movements that achieve the same thing. Older people don't heal as fast as younger people. Don't try to see how much weight you can lift – unless you want to support your local orthopedic surgeon. Taking time off to recover from injuries defeats your purpose. I've made more gains using *Time & Retention* with moderate weight than I ever did using maximum weight and low reps.

Get good weight lifting gloves with wrap-around wrist support. Buy Thorlo socks for maximum cushion against foot problems, to prevent shin splints, promote optimal wicking (moisture management)

and for protection from blis-
ters (see Suppliers
Directory). Wear a good
warm-up suit to start, then
remove after warming up.
Eat some low-glycemic
carbs before working out;
during workouts your
muscles need the energy.
Minimize socializing – concentrate on workouts – and move fast
between sets. Keep workouts to an hour or

Thorlo socks unique cushion design prevent, or cures shin splints and protects your feet. I wear them as my daily socks and when exercising.

less (except leg day, which can be longer). Fatigued muscles need protein soon after working out. Eat a protein supplement 15-20 minutes
after lifting. Supplements reach your fatigued muscles fast, whereas
regular food can take hours.

Two-thirds of the body's total muscle is below the waist. When
you work legs hard, you need time to recover. Always take the day off
after leg day to rest.

The sample workout plan in the following chapter is excellent for
a fat-to-muscle transition, although there are many different routines
to accomplish the same thing. Adjust workouts for your somatotype
and weaknesses. For instance, if you have weak triceps or calves,
work them twice a week instead of once. To avoid over training, work
each major body part directly only once per week.

Those of you trying to lose body fat should weight train 3-5 days
a week and do 20-30 minutes of aerobic exercise three times a week,
depending how overfat you are. Utilize the unique *Time & Retention*
weight training techniques to make gains fast and reduce chances of
injury.

Free Weights vs. Machines

Weight lifters have long favored free weights (dumbbells and barbells) over machines. This is because free weights utilize more muscle fibers to balance the weights. Today, however, many of the new
machines are excellent for targeting certain muscle groups.

Using machines, especially for *Time & Retention*, it is often easier and safer to control the negative, or downward, movement when
lowering the weight. This is the part of the movement that should be
slower and controlled. Weights can be lowered with little resistance,

whereas machines and cables require a slower, controlled descent. The lowering of the weight is where you will achieve most of the muscle hypertrophy that results in increased strength and growth.

Examples of *Time & Retention* exercises that can be done with machines include seated leg extensions, hamstring curls, leg presses, Smith bar squats and lunges, seated lat cable pulls, lat pull downs and calf raises.

Hire A Personal Trainer

An experienced personal trainer will show you many things – hand positions, breathing and different lifts and routines – all techniques to help you make gains faster. A trainer can customize workouts, diets and supplements for your somatotype. A good trainer will also help keep you motivated and focused. Some trainers specialize in injury recovery, and can help you deal with new or chronic injuries.

Interview trainers who have a physique similar to what you desire. Does the trainer exhibit good listening skills and communicate well? Is the trainer certified through a nationally recognized organization (APEX, ACE, ACSM, NASM or equivalent)? Is the trainer serious about getting results, or is the club policy "Don't make anybody sore or they won't come back?"

It is one thing to read a book and pass a test and another to actually do it. Avoid "book smart" trainers. Find a lean, muscular trainer. They know the secret to losing fat, getting fit and gaining muscle. Let your trainer know you are serious and expect results. Do your part – eat right and don't miss workouts.

Many fitness clubs utilize a computer-aided program that analyzes your specific fitness goals and considers your age, injuries, and food preferences. The Apex program, available in many gyms, is one of the best. You fill out a questionnaire and the computer prints out a customized exercise, diet and supplement program for you. It's an excellent format for trainers to follow because it eliminates guesswork. When a gym uses an Apex program, the trainers are Apex certified to interpret your individual diet and exercise needs and to help you follow and stick with the program. *Spend the money for a trainer, it's for your body and it's one of the best investments you'll ever make.*

Weight Training Routine

This is an excellent routine for a fat-to-muscle transition. Hire a trainer to teach you the proper technique of all exercises, as technique cannot be shown in photos. Adjust routines and workouts to meet somatotype and goals. Utilize **Time & Retention** *wherever possible.*

Day 1:   **Chest, triceps, calves**
Day 2:   **Rest**
Day 3:   **Legs, abs**
Day 4:   **Rest**
Day 5:   **Deltoids, traps, abs**
Day 6:   **Back, biceps**
Day 7:   **Rest**
Day 8:   **Cycle begins again**

Day 1   Chest, Triceps, Calves

CHEST

Warm up using cable flyes doing a set of 25-35 reps with light weight. Stretch.

Cable flyes: One set. Using work weight, do four or five reps, then hold together touching palms of hands for 25-35 seconds or failure.

Dumbbell or machine flat, incline, and decline presses: One set of each with bench set at 30 degrees raised, 30 degrees lowered and flat. Do a few reps, then hold each for 25-30 seconds or failure. (Have a spotter when using dumbbells.)

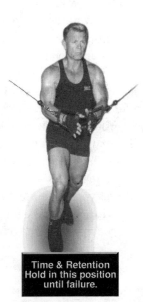

Time & Retention
Hold in this position
until failure.

TRICEPS

Warm up set of 25-35 with light weight. Stretch.

Bent-over tricep presses: *Do a few full range of motion reps, then move dumb-bells to raised point at top of movement and hold for 25-35 seconds or failure.*

Triceps push downs: *One set. Keeping elbows close to side, don't go higher than 90 degrees. Do a few full range of motion reps, then hold at 90 degrees for 25-35 seconds or failure.*

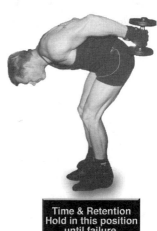

Time & Retention
Hold in this position
until failure.

CALVES

Standing calf raises: *Three sets, each work set of 18 reps pyramiding up in weight. Work on full range of motion. Go all the way down as far as possible and all the way up your toes. Hold last set in raised position for 25-35 seconds to failure.*

Seated calf raises: *Three sets of 18 using same technique.*

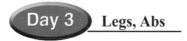

Day 3 **Legs, Abs**

LEGS *(legs are your largest muscle group)*

Warm up with 25-35 leg presses using one-third of your work weight. You can use heavy weight on work set. Most people don't real-ize how strong their legs are.

Leg presses: *Do a few reps, then hold weight in weakest contracted position for 25-35 seconds or failure.*

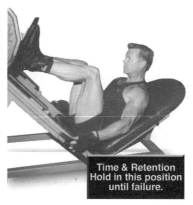

Time & Retention
Hold in this position
until failure.

Hamstring curls: *Warm up with 25-35 reps using light weight. Do either lying or seated hamstring curls. Do a few reps and hold in contracted position for 25-35 seconds or failure.*

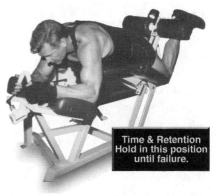

Time & Retention
Hold in this position
until failure.

Leg extensions: *Do a few reps, then hold in contracted position for 25-35 seconds or failure.*

Adductor machine: *Do a few reps, then hold in contracted position for 25-35 seconds to failure.*

ABDOMINALS

Incline sit ups: *Adjust bench height for your fitness level. Do a few, then hold in halfway up position with hands folded over chest.*

Rope pull downs: *Three sets. Go all the way down touching elbows, squeeze abs at bottom for 1 second, return to top of movement. Don't jerk, go up slower than you go down. You should feel a good burn; if not, increase weight.*

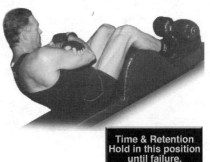

Time & Retention
Hold in this position
until failure.

Day 5   Deltoids, traps, abs

Important Note: Rotator and shoulder problems are common weight training injuries. Always warm up the shoulders with the following exercise and avoid straight bar bench presses.

Dumbbell raises: *(5 lbs. or less) Do a set of 25-35, then stretch.*

DELTOIDS

Warm up set of 25-35 dumbbell raises with one dumbbell using light weight. Stretch.

Front Dumbbell Lift: *Using one dumbbell, do three sets, pyramiding up in weight. Do a few reps and then hold the dumbbell with arms straight in front, shoulder level, for 25-35 seconds or failure.*

Dumbbell Raises: *Three sets of dumbbell raises side, front and under chin. Using light weight, do three sets of 8-15 reps for each position, with no rest between each position.*

Traps: *Do three sets dumbbell shrugs. Do a few reps and then hold in contracted position for 25-35 seconds or failure.*

Time & Retention
Hold in this position
until failure.

ABDOMINALS

Do three sets of rope pull downs working up in weight each set. Focus on form, using only your abs to pull, not your back. Hold at the bottom squeez-ing your abs for 1 second, touching your elbows. Go all the way up, don't jerk.

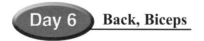

Day 6 | **Back, Biceps**

Important Note: *Use light weight. A 175-lb. man should use about 60 pounds. Adjust your work weight to your fitness level. Stretch between sets.*

Lat pull-downs: *Do three sets (each set is 15-15-15) following this format. Do 15 with hands wide, palms awa,. 15 with hands close, palms facing you, 15 with palms away shoulder width. Do not rest between changing hand positions for each 15. Rest two minutes between sets.*

Bar or machine pull-ups: *Do three sets. Do a few reps, then hold position with chin at bar level for 25-35 seconds or failure. (If you can't do pull ups, use a weight assisted pull up machine). These are tough, but they are the best total back workout.*

Machine or cable rows: *Do one set. Do a few reps, then hold for 25-35 seconds or failure.*

BICEPS
Warm up with 25-35 standing dumbbell curls. Stretch.

Machine bicep curls: *Do three sets. Pyramiding up in weight, do a few reps, then hold for 25-35 seconds or failure.*

Seated dumbbell curls: *Do one set. Do a few reps alternating arms to touch chest , then hold dumbbells in 90 degree position for 25-35 seconds to failure.*

Standing cable curls: *Do a few reps, then hold for 30-40 seconds to failure.*

chapter 36

Home Gyms

Are home gyms as effective as going to the gym? No…but there are many advantages to having a home gym. You save the driving time; you can work out before you shower; you don't have the initial fees or monthly dues and you'll probably use the home gym more because of the convenience factor.

According to American Sports Data Inc., of the 53 million who strength train at home, only 8 million use home gyms. Looking to capture a larger share of the ever-growing baby boomer market, manufacturers have made significant improvements in the last year.

These new "multidirectional resistance" home gyms now allow movements that mimic free weights by providing movements that don't lock your movements into a prescribed path. Similar to dumbbells, you must use supporting muscles to balance the weight even as the prime movers do their work. They are more compact, feature more

Powerblocks are great for home gyms because they replace a full set of dumbbells in a two foot space.

exercise options, are durable, affordable and safe to use. Prices range from $1500-$2350.

I have a set of Powerblocks in my home gym which eliminate the need for a full rack of dumb-bells. You simply add or sub-tract weight by use of a pin. Powerblock's adjustable bench enables you to do a wide variety of exercises for all body parts except heavy leg work. I also have a seated Ab Bench which I've found is the best

The Ab Bench is great for home gyms. The movement it provides builds strong abdom-inals fast.

machine for hitting the abdominals. Because abdominals are muscles that respond to weight resistance, the Ab Bench is far superior than doing crunches.

These home gyms will never replace the variety the local gym offers, but they do provide good work-outs if you learn how to use them properly. I usually work legs at the gym but often use my home gym for other body parts because of the convenience factor.

Several popular home gyms include Bowflex, Hoist, Nordictrack, Powertec, Body-Solid, Parabody and Pacific Fitness.

I use a bowflex in my home gym because it provides all the basic exe-cises with ample weight. It also works great for Time & Resistan because, unlike dumbbells, you can't just drop the weight.

❓ Fiction

If you perform "normal" range of motion weight lifting exer-cises you'll never have injuries.

❗ Fact

*Joint and tendon injuries from normal weight lifting is only a matter of time. **Time & Retention** weight lifting will lower chances of injuries and you'll make faster gains.*

chapter 37 Step 4: Aerobic Exercise

We all rely on the beating of our hearts but not all of our hearts beat efficiently. The resting heart rate (RHR), of the average adult human beats about 72 times per minute. The heart of a well-trained aerobic athlete beats as slowly as 35 times per minute.

The "Golden Rule" of aerobic exercise is that you sustain an elevated pulse rate of approximately 65-75% of your maximum heart rate (MHR). What is the average MHR at age 50? MHR is 220 beats per minute minus age. That puts average 50-year-old people at about 170. This would make your "target" heart rate about 110 (65% of 170). However, this formula doesn't apply to everyone usually (but not always), conditioned athletes have much lower heart rates.

For example, Bjorn Borg had an RHR of 35 beats-per-minute (BPM). This makes sense; Borg was an elite tennis player. But Olympic marathoner Frank Shorter's RHR was 75 BPM. Genes account for about 50% of what resting heart rate will turn out to be. Smaller hearts beat faster than larger ones. In general, the more fit you are, the stronger your heart beat (stroke volume).

The average RHR for women is 78-84 beats per minute and 72-78 for men. Does your heart beat faster or slower than average? Check the following chart for your target heart rate. We older athletes should target the lower end because our muscles take longer to recover. You should be able to carry on a conversation, not gasping for breath, during your aerobic exercise. If you're working too hard, you're working "anaerobically", which means you're not effectively burning body fat.

You should be in the "target zone" halfway through your workout. Check your heart rate by placing your index and middle fingers over the artery on the underside of your wrist, applying light pressure. Count ten seconds and multiply the number of beats by 6. This tells you your current heart rate. You should check your heart rate periodically to make sure you're in your target zone, and increase or decrease your workout accordingly.

Do aerobic exercise first thing in the morning to avoid muscle loss and promote fat loss. This is much more important than how long you do aerobic exercise. Doing aerobic exercise first thing in the morning suppresses insulin levels, liberating free fatty acids for energy. This "jump starts" your metabolism and gets you going for the entire day. *In order to optimally burn body fat you should have an empty stomach.* No calories, only water, should be consumed prior to your morning training. This forces your body to burn fat stores for energy.

Figure Your "Target" Heartrate

Age	Target HR Zone 50-75% beats per min.	Avg. Max. HR HR 100%
20	100-150	200
25	98-146	195
30	95-142	190
35	93-138	185
40	90-135	180
45	88-131	175
50	85-127	170
55	83-123	165
60	80-120	160
65	78-116	155
70	75-113	150

Your maximum heart rate is approximately 220 minus your age. The figures above are averages and should be used as general guidelines.

Your morning exercise should be 20 minutes of medium intensity training. Eat breakfast immediately after your morning exercise. Your body will now digest food more effectively with little chance of storing any excess calories as body fat.

Sedentary people (those who can't run around the block) should start by brisk walking. You can then move up to walking hills, then jogging. Those in decent shape (capable of running one mile) should start with 65% of their MHR. Elite athletes in good shape (capable of running three miles), should start with 75%of their MHR for 20 minutes. As you improve, add six 30-60 second wind sprints, spaced evenly throughout the session.

If possible, runners should stick to asphalt, avoiding concrete sidewalks or roads. Asphalt provides more cushion and is easier on the feet and joints. Also, avoid surfaces that aren't level, like high crested roads, running paths and beaches. A sloping surface is very hard on the joints and feet. Those with existing foot problems or old injuries should consult a podiatrist for special orthotics for running.

If you don't have the time to do aerobic exercise in the morning, the next best time to do it is immediately after you weight train. Your body will have used most of its fuel calories (glycogen) during the weight lifting session since carbohydrates are the preferred fuels for intense work. When you start your aerobic session after lifting, you will be using fat as fuel. If you do aerobics before lifting, your body burns calories consumed from your last meal as energy, not stored body fat.

If you can't do aerobics in the morning or after weight training, the next best time is immediately before going to bed. This will increase your metabolic rate not only while you're doing it, but into your sleeping hours as well. Do not eat after this session; this will help to prevent food being stored as body fat while sleeping. Adjust aerobic routines to your individual goals and fitness levels. As you exercise, your cardiovascular system will get stronger to keep up with the demands of your body. After just a few weeks, you'll be pumping more blood per beat. This will reduce your resting and working heart rate.

The best aerobic exercises are those that incorporate legs and arms, such as running, rowing, cross country skiing and circuit weight training. You burn more calories using arms and legs simultaneously. For example, when walking on a non-motorized treadmill with an arm exerciser, you'll burn an average of 900 calories per hour at 3 mph; while walking without arm exercise at the same pace you'll burn 600 calories per hour. You'll get a one-third increase by using your arms as well as your legs.

chapter 38

Step 5: Do We Need Supplements?

very day a war is being waged on our immune systems. Never before in the history of medicine has the well-being of our immune systems been so important, as it is our immune systems that protect our health and longevity. Antibiotic resistant bacteria and strange, virulent viruses that have defied all of medicine's attempts to eradicate them are now a fact of life – or death!

I don't know how many times I've heard "I get all the nutrients I need by eating healthy." Need for what? Everyone should consider using supplements to stay healthy. Weight lifters need to supplement to maximize gains and maintain energy levels. During ketosis, supplementing is essential to get the nutrients eliminated by calorie reduction (CR).

Daily pollution, smoke, chemicals, stress, exercis, and other toxins produce substances called free radicals. Free radicals are chemical by-products of oxygen metabolism that attack cell components and irreversibly damage them. They also contribute to aging and disease. Free radicals cause imbalances in our immune systems, making us more vulnerable to cardiovascular disease, cancer, prostate problems and many other diseases.

Our immune systems protect us against free radicals and other diseases from outside sources and within our bodies. It goes after viruses, yeast, fungus and bacteria. It seeks and destroys cancer cells. It even involves itself in digestion when necessary. It plays an integral role in healing and is greatly involved in inflammation, asthma, allergies and psoriasis.

When the immune system becomes overloaded, without proper nutrition, it may become confused and attack the body itself. This may explain why Americans are facing an ever-increasing onset of autoimmune diseases, including rheumatoid arthritis, lupus, multiple sclerosis, fibromyalgia and Crohn's disease.

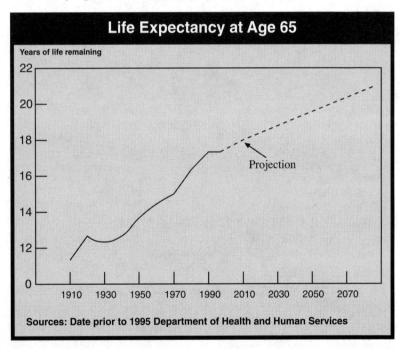

Life Expectancy at Age 65

Years of life remaining

Projection

Sources: Date prior to 1995 Department of Health and Human Services

Life expectancy in America should be 85-90 years of age and living to 100 should be considered normal. There are many primitive people around the world today whose life expectancies are much greater than Americans and they don't have the modern medical support we do.

These societies are rarely overfat, are strong, muscular and they don't suffer the ravages of old age such as increased blood pressure, cancer, atherosclerosis and lowered immune systems like Americans.

They get essential minerals in the high glacier mountain water they drink, they do not eat processed foods and physical labor is a

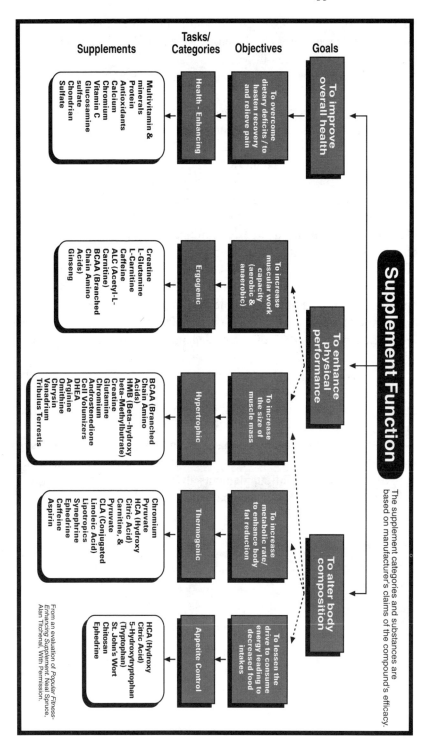

Supplement Function

The supplement categories and substances are based on manufacturer's claims of the compound's efficacy.

Supplements	Tasks/Categories	Objectives	Goals
Multivitamin & minerals, Protein, Antioxidants, Calcium, Chromium, Vitamin C, Glucosamine sulfate, Chondrian Sulfate	Health - Enhancing	To overcome dietary deficits / to hasten recovery and relieve pain	To improve overall health
Creatine, L-Glutamine, L-Carnitine, Caffeine, ALC (Acetyl-L-Carnitine), BCAA (Branched Chain Amino Acids), Ginseng	Ergogenic	To increase muscular work capacity (aerobic & anaerobic)	To enhance physical performance
BCAA (Branched Chain Amino Acids), HMB (Beta-hydroxy beta-Methylbutrate), Creatine, Glutamine, Chromium, Androstenedione, DHEA, Cell Volumizers, Arginine, Ornitine, Chrysin, Vanadrium, Tribulus Terrestis	Hypertrophic	To increase the size of muscle mass	
Chromium, Pyruvate, HCA (Hydroxy Citric Acid), Carnitine, & Pyruvate, CLA (Conjugated Linoleic Acid), Lipotropics, Synephrine, Ephedrine, Caffeine, Aspirin	Thermogenic	To increase metabolic rate/ to enhance body fat reduction	To alter body composition
HCA (Hydroxy Citric Acid), 5-Hydroxytryptophan (Tryptophan), St. John's Wort, Chitosan, Ephedrine	Appetite Control	To lessen the drive to consume energy leading to decreased food intakes	

From an evaluation of *Popular Fitness-Enhancing Supplement.* Neal Spruce, Alan Titcheral, With Permission.

daily part of their lives. Even though these people often die of infection in infancy or early childhood, if we adopt their living habits, we could have the best of both worlds!

There are several supplements that are essential to good health, longevity and maximizing muscle gains while losing body fat. You should consider supplementing long term, but it is especially important during your 90 day fat-to-muscle transition. When you stop eating "junk food", you eliminate the "empty" calories – fat and sugar – but you also lose essential nutrients. Training hard requires even more nutrients for energy and recovery. Supplements provide the nutrients you need without empty calories you don't need.

If you supplement, does that mean you don't have to eat right? Humans have relied on food for millions of years. There has never been a successful attempt to keep an animal or person healthy – or even alive – on a diet composed strictly of nutritional supplements. Supplementing alone is an inadequate and incomplete method of supplying nutrients, as it is impossible to match nature's refined balances.

Experts agree there are at least 100,000 nutrients. Scientists have identified only 10-40% of them, depending on what authority you believe.

This is why food should be the most important element and the very foundation of any nutritional program. Supplements are just what the name implies – an additional back up for sound nutrition to maximize gains. They aren't a magic bullet or the fountain of youth.

In the following chapters I have explained the best – and worst – supplements. Take only those supplements that have been tested and proven to work. Avoid supplements that may have negative health effects, or have no proven medical value.

Fiction
There is no reason to supplement if we eat healthy.

Fact
It's nearly impossible to eat enough of the right foods to get the nutrients we need for optimal health and longevity. Athletes need even more nutrients than sedentary people.

chapter 39

The Best Vitamins & Minerals

E ven if we ate our government's RDA of food, we wouldn't be getting the important nutrients we need to stay healthy and certainly not enough to build muscle and extend our longevity. When we exercise, especially with weights, we create more damaging free radicals than sedentary people do.

Antioxidants neutralize microscopic "free radicals" and are found in the best vitamin-mineral supplements. They occur naturally in the body and can also be obtained from certain foods. The top ten foods high in antioxidants are berries, broccoli, tomatoes, red grapes, garlic, spinach, tea, carrots, soy and whole grains. Why, then, don't we just eat these plants and skip the supplements?

Even if we did eat enough of these plants (15-20 per day in the right combination), we probably wouldn't get the essential nutrients we need. That's because our food doesn't contain the nutrients it did in paleo times. For millions of years our caveman ancestors ate foods rich in vitamins and minerals from virgin soil. In fact, their vitamin-mineral consumption was much higher than what our government recommends we eat today.

NUTRIENT	PALEOLITHIC INTAKE	RDA
Vitamin C	600 mg	60 mg
Vitamin E	33 mg	8-10 mg
Calicum	2000 mg	800-1200 mg
Magnesium	700 mg	350 mg
Potassium	10,000 mg	3,500 mg
Zinc	43 mg	12-15 mg
Fiber	50-100 grams	25-35 grams

Paleolithic man got more of every nutrient than we do, sometimes much more.

We inherited our early ancestor's biochemistry. The great variety of minerals present in their food for millions of years resulted in the mineral dependency of our bodies. When it comes to the minerals we need, the problem is even greater because plants cannot make minerals. If the minerals aren't in the soils, the plants can't make vitamins. *It only takes 5-10 years to pull the nutrients out of the soil.* Today's intense farming and overpopulation have depleted our soils of the minerals and nutrients we need to stay healthy.

According to Senate Document 264, "The alarming fact is that foods (fruits, vegetables and grains) now being raised on millions of acres of the land that no longer contain enough of certain minerals are starving us – no matter how much of them we eat. No man of today can eat enough fruits and vegetables to supply his system with the minerals he requires for perfect health, because his stomach isn't big enough to hold them." This warning was issued in 1936 and the situation has only worsened since then!

Even though nitrogen, phosphorus and potassium are added to the soil to grow larger plants, this doesn't add the minerals back to the soil. Many farmers grow genetically altered crops with high levels of test tube toxins, sprayed with GMO compatible herbicides, to grow large, sweet fruits and "hopped up" vegetables that are often devoid of the basic nutrients we need.

Joel Wallach B.S., D.V.M, N.D. is one of the country's leading authorities on nutrition and mineral deficiency diseases. Being raised on a farm, he learned first hand how vitamins and minerals are mixed into livestock feed in order to keep the livestock healthy.

Dr. Wallach became a veterinarian and performed over 17,500 autopsies on over 454 species of animals which died of "natural" causes at the St. Louis, Brookfield, Los Angeles and Bronx Zoos. He later became a doctor and performed over 3,000 autopsies on humans who died of "natural" causes. What he discovered was that *every animal and human that died of "natural" causes actually died of a nutritional deficiency.*

Dr. Wallach then started research projects in which he gave humans supplements. The nutritional supplements had profound effects on humans. His twelve year study showed that humans stayed healthier and lived longer, just like the farm and zoo animals, when they were supplementing. According to Wallach, we need 90 nutrients, in optimal amounts, in our daily diet to prevent a deficiency disease. This includes 60 minerals, 16 vitamins, 12 essential amino acids or protein building blocks and 3 essential fatty acids.

It is not uncommon for dogs to live 15 years or longer. That's 105 years old in "people years". Why do dogs live so long? Because companies like Purina put around 40 vitamins and minerals in their dog food. Have you noticed dogs get sick a lot less than humans? *There are no human infant formulas that have more than 11 minerals!*

Liquids vs. Hard Capsules

According to the *Physician's Desk Reference*, considered the "Medical Bible" for doctors, our bodies absorb no more than 10-20% of most nutrients in pill form, compared to 98% of liquids. The scenario is even worse because older people absorb less than half the amount of minerals than younger people do.

Does your urine turn bright yellow after taking your daily multiple? This means that for every $100 you spend on nutrients in pill form, you're flushing at least $80 down the toilet!

Metallic minerals like oyster shells, carbonates, oxides and dolomites have the consistency of crushed rock, which our bodies cannot digest. Even pills listed as "all natural" often have added fillers and coatings that inhibit absorption.

Supplementing with a quality liquid multiple containing vitamins, minerals, antioxidants, phytonutrients and botanical extracts will substantially fortify your immune system to prevent damage from free radicals.

Liquid multiples provide a 98% absorption rate because they bypass the digestive process and go directly into the blood stream and

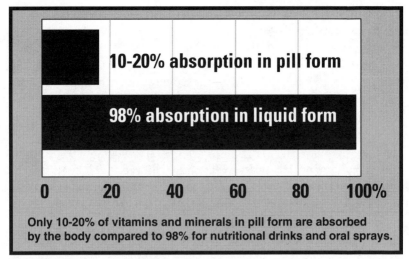

10-20% absorption in pill form

98% absorption in liquid form

0   20   40   60   80   100%

Only 10-20% of vitamins and minerals in pill form are absorbed by the body compared to 98% for nutritional drinks and oral sprays.

Physician's Desk Reference, page 1542

into the cells within a matter of minutes. Liquids are much faster and easier to take. Liquids don't cause the problems that pills do, including irritable bowel syndrome, hiatal hernias and diverticulitis.

Liquid multiples can also help lower and normalize blood sugar to prevent fat gain. Blood work tests have also shown that liquid multiples often improve high cholesterol levels and cancer. Blood work is the most objective proof we have.

Take an all natural liquid multiple that contains the major vitamins, trace minerals, enzymes, amino acids and botanical extracts...all essential nutrients that are missing from the average diet.

Calcium

Osteoporosis is a disease that affects millions of Americans each year. Most people in the U.S. are consuming 60% or less of the calcium RDA. (I agree with the RDA on this one.) Calcium comes in many different salt forms. Calcium citrate mallet has the highest rate of absorption.

Calcium dosages suggested for nutritional adequacy differ depending on age and sex. From ages 25 to 50, the RDA is 1000mg. Post-menopausal women should consume 1500 mg. People who exercise lose calcium in their sweat. Those on high protein diets also require additional calcium. It is therefore important to supplement calcium on the *Muscle & Longevity* program and these supplements should be taken with meals.

chapter 40

The Power Of Protein

Protein supplements help build muscle and curb appetite. ***Eating protein every few hours is essential for a fat-to-muscle transition.*** There are a large variety of excellent protein supplements from which to choose, including whey, soy and whey-peptide blends.

There are three criterion for selecting a protein supplement including "biological value" (BV), protein efficiency ration (PER) and protein digestibility corrected amino acid score (PDCAAS). The biological value scale (how many usable grams it contains) was developed using an egg as a basis – an egg being 100%. Fish has 83% and beef has 80%.

Protein Source	RATING METHODS			
	B.V.	P.E.R.	N.P.U.	PDCAAS
Whey Protein	104	3.6	92	1.0
Whole Egg	100	3.8	94	1.0
Beef	80	2.0	73	0.92
Casein (milk)	77	2.9	76	1.0
Soy	74	2.1	61	0.99
Rice	59	2.0	57	0.26
Beans	49	1.4	39	0.68

Research shows that whey protein is actually improved by combining sources when processed under the right conditions, creating unique bio-active growth factors. That's why whey peptide blends, with a rating of 110-159%, are the best source of protein supplements.

Find a protein that tastes good and is formulated to yield slow releasing carbohydrates. Avoid protein supplements with aspartame, phenylalanine, partially hydrogenated vegetable oil, maltodextrin (a 100+ on the glycemic index) or artificial flavors.

Instead of high glycemic sugar substitutes like maltodextrin, some modern protein supplements use low glycemic sugar replacements ,including crystalline fructose and fruit extracts. These new protein supplements taste good and contain a wide variety of micro-nutrients, vitamins and minerals, glutamine and other metabolic support nutrients.

Protein can be put in a blender with water and ice to make shakes or can be mixed with water. Some come in single serving plastic bottles, which can be filled with water and shaken – a real convenience for those on the go. Avoid protein bars when "cutting" body fat. They all contain a lot of sugar and/or more fat than a jelly donut.

Because the amino acids in protein cannot be stored, eating large amounts of protein at one meal won't work. Eating protein every few hours prevents the body from regressing to a catabolic state, burning muscle for energy and keeps blood sugar levels stable.

Protein reduces your appetite for sweets, which cause insulin surges, in turn facilitating fat storage. A protein supplement should be eaten in the morning between breakfast and lunch, in the afternoon between lunch and dinner and immediately after working out in the evening. Every three hours, men can assimilate 35-40 grams of protein and women can assimilate 20-25 grams.

Ideal Weight	DAILY PROTEIN SUGGESTIONS			
	Minimum	Medium	Typical	Bodybuilder
	0.34g/lb.	0.5g/lb.	1g/lb.	1.3g/lb.
80 lbs.	27g	40g	80g	104g
100 lbs.	34g	50g	100g	130g
120 lbs.	41g	60g	120g	156g
140 lbs.	48g	70g	140g	182g
160 lbs.	54g	80g	160g	208g
180 lbs.	61g	90g	180g	234g
200 lbs.	68g	100g	200g	260g
220 lbs.	75g	110g	220g	286g

chapter 41

Creatine Monohydrate

Creatine is one of the muscle's main energy sources. Creatine is a natural nutrient found in varying quantities in a variety of foods. The food source with the highest amount of creatine is red meat, with approximately 5 grams in 2.2 pounds. Supplementing creatine gives us this important nutrient that we need to build lean muscle, without the fat and calories from meat sources.

Because 95% of creatine is stored inside muscle cells, creatine monohydrate induces cell volumizing. Cellular hydration is a major control point for protein metabolism. Muscle cell swelling stimulates the synthesis of protein and therefore an increased cell volume can mimic certain hormones' positive effects on protein metabolism. Cell hydration during weight training leads to an increase in muscle tissue.

Creatine is especially effective for middle aged people. Research has shown aging is associated with a decline in muscle phosphocreatine levels. This is probably because middle aged people have less fast-twitch muscle fibers than younger people. These type II fast twitch fibers store most of the creatine that muscles require for energy.

Recent creatine supplementation research on younger men, compared to men 50 and older, showed resting phosphocreatine increased

15% in the younger group and 30% in the middle aged group.

Furthermore, the older group also increased their ability to re-synthesize phosphocreatine by about 30%. Creatine supplementation increased muscle endurance and delayed fatigue twice as much in older people.

Creatine increases strength, enabling the muscles to recover faster. This results in more rapid increases in lean muscle and reduction of body fat, which is why creatine is one of the best supplements for older folks who lift weights. Take 5 grams per day (skip the loading phase) for 3 weeks, then take 2 weeks off. Take creatine with water 45 minutes before weight lifting so it will be in your system, working, when your muscles need it.

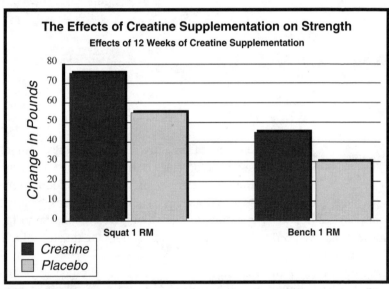

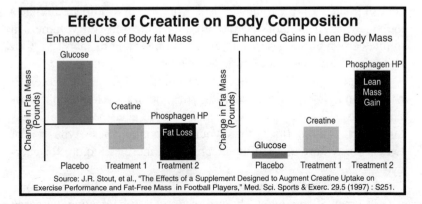

Source: J.R. Stout, et al., "The Effects of a Supplement Designed to Augment Creatine Uptake on Exercise Performance and Fat-Free Mass in Football Players," Med. Sci. Sports & Exerc. 29.5 (1997) : S251.

chapter 42 **Carnitine – Slows The Aging Process**

A s more research is done, Carnitine (completely natural and non-toxic), has emerged as one of the most important nutrients for slowing the natural aging process. As body levels of carnitine – our main energizing nutrient – decline as we age, our cells are not as energetic. Energy is the greatest anti-aging force known. A decrease in cellular energy is the main reason the aging process actually accelerates as we grow older. Carnitine and acetyl-L-carnitine (a special form of carnitine) can help slow down the aging process.

It is especially important to supplement carnitine when losing body fat by ketosis. Carnitine helps the liver make blood sugar from protein in the diet, a process called gluconeogenesis. This will eliminate fatigue or headaches that can sometimes occur in ketosis. Carnitine ensures that energy levels will remain high by helping the body adjust from burning mostly carbohydrates to burning fat for energy.

As we age, our bodies are less capable of protecting us from free radicals. Carnitine also helps protect cells from damage when fighting free radicals and fortifies the immune system, especially as we age. Both carnitine and acetyl-L-carnitine boost our free radical defenses and help create a better balance of fats in the blood and cells. This helps prevent heart disease and reduces the chances of contracting diseases associated with inflammation.

Circulation and oxygen levels slow down with age. With less oxygen to live on, cells make less energy and die, which results in premature aging. Carnitine protects against this and allows cells to recover from the damage that occurs due to lack of oxygen levels in tissues.

Acetyl-L-carnitine levels in the brain decline with age, causing deterioration of brain cells. Acetyl-L-carnitine has the particular ability to optimize brain function and prevent this deterioration. It acts as a powerful antioxidant and substantially increases levels of an important messenger molecule called acetylcholine, while providing the brain with healing energy. After age 40, acetyl-L-carnitine is the preferred form of carnitine.

Fiction
There is no supplement that will slow the aging process.

Fact
Acetyl-L-Carnitine has nutrients which help slow the natural aging process.

chapter 43 **Glucosamine &**
Chondroitin Sulfates

C artilage is slowly lost in joints with age or injury. Because cartilage acts as a lubricant, its loss causes friction and pain. To make up for this decrease in lubrication, synovial fluid is excreted from the synovium (the joint lining). Although this slick substance increases lubrication, it can cause swelling and pain if present in large amounts.

Glucosamine sulfate is a naturally occurring mucopolysaccharide found in certain seafood products. Glucosamine and chondroitin are integral substrates in cartilage metabolism. *Both have been shown to have beneficial effects in reducing pain and increasing mobility.*

Proteoglycans in glucosamine sulfate attract water to the joint and provide essential lubrication. Many studies compare glucosamine to ibuprofen, which is commonly used to treat inflammatory pain. In research studies, both were equal in pain treatment but glucosamine had fewer side effects.

I've found glucosamine and chondroitin sulfate most effective, but it takes about six weeks to start working. Nearly everyone I've recommended it to reports their joint pain has disappeared or improved significantly. I take it every day.

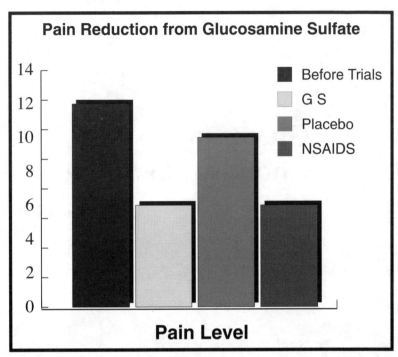

Pain Reduction from Glucosamine Sulfate

Legend:
- Before Trials
- G S
- Placebo
- NSAIDS

Y-axis: 0, 2, 4, 6, 8, 10, 12, 14

X-axis: Pain Level

Glucosamine Sulfate is effective for reducing joint pain, a common injury for weight lifters.

Fiction
Only aspirin or Ibuprofen can stop joint pain.

Fact
Glucosamine and chondroitin have proven beneficial effects in reducing joint pain.

chapter 44

Natural Sex Supplements

N early 80% of men ages 30-80 will experience a decreased sex drive or difficulty in getting or maintaining an erection at sometime. In America, 18% of men are impotent by the age of 60 and the same percentage of women lose their sexual drive.

The popular drug, Viagra, is reported to have amazing effects on enhancing libido. The magic "blue bullet", however, does have a few drawbacks, including side effects, the need for a prescription and high cost per dose.

Although nothing improves libido like getting fit, recent research has proven many natural compounds that don't require a prescription can greatly enhance many sexual functions. Unlike their pharmaceutical cousins, they have other health benefits, including the ability to help build muscle. Even if you don't have a problem but just want a stronger sex drive or to enhance your performance, these supplements can take your sex life from ordinary to incredible.

The best-proven natural compounds include Arginine, Yohimbine and Ginkgo Biloba. Of these, Yohimbine, which comes from the bark of the African Yohimbe tree, tops the list. Yohimbe HCL is marketed as a supplement for sexual dysfunction and has a growing number of scientific studies to support it. Unlike many "aphrodisiac" compounds, the mechanisms by which yohimbine works have been well documented and proven.

Yohimbine can improve sex several ways. Yohimbine helps increase penile blood inflow and decreases penile blood outflow. The results are obvious – getting more blood to the penis and keeping it there provides for a larger and longer lasting erection. Plus, yohimbine temporarily blocks the sympathetic nervous system. This helps prevent male premature ejaculation, increasing the duration of intercourse. Not a bad aerobic workout, when you consider you can burn up to 400 calories with thirty minutes of sex!

Yohimbine is also a mild stimulant (some people actually report being over-stimulated), which results in more energy and burns more body fat. There are a few things to know before rushing out and buying this product. People on MAOI's (monoamine oxidase inhibitors) or those with heart disease, high blood pressure, diabetes or liver disease usually feel excessive stimulation from this compound and shouldn't take it. If you take any prescription drugs and want to try Yohimbine, check with your physician and pharmacist, as there are certain medications that can interact.

Arginine is rapidly growing as a popular sex aid. Arginine is a precursor necessary for the production of nitric oxide, which signals the body to relax the smooth muscle tissue of the penis. As these smooth muscles relax, blood flows into the penis and it becomes erect. In many ways arginine provides similar, although less as powerful, effects as Viagra.

Arginine also aides muscle growth because it stimulates growth hormone release. Arginine is good for the heart, due to its ability to lower cholesterol. It also improves wound healing and increases sperm mobility in men. Arginine has virtually no toxicity, few contraindications with prescription drugs and is inexpensive. If you decide to use arginine, look for products that recommend dosages of about 2 grams.

Ginkgo Biloba has long been recognized for its positive effect on libido as well as for its excellent antioxidant properties. Ginkgo helps protect capillaries, due to its antioxidant functions. This, in turn, supports a critical part of the process that leads to erection. Most people also experience improved energy levels when using ginkgo.

The only potential problem for using ginkgo is that it may thin blood. This means that people already using blood-thinning medication, such as Coumadin, should consult with their physician prior to taking any supplement containing ginkgo. There are several other

herbs that have long been touted as aphrodisiacs and are now marketed as alternatives to Viagra. The problem is that little or no research
regarding their efficacy or safety has been done. These include Horny
Goat Weed, Tribulous, Maca and Epimedium, to name a few. I would
advise avoiding supplements with these ingredients until more
research has been done on them.

Based on the research and cost/benefit ratio, find a product that
contains arginine, yohimbine and ginkgo biloba. I'd also suggest saw
palmetto, especially for those with prostate trouble. Look for stan-
dardized herbal extracts that guarantee the actual constituents necessary for optimal results.

❓ Fiction
Viagra is the best cure for impotency.

❗ Fact
*Nothing improves libido like getting fit, but there are many
natural compounds that help.*

chapter 45

Stimulants & Thermogenics

C offee and tea both contain caffeine, but the amount found in a cup doesn't pose a long-term health problem for most people. It can be beneficial to drink coffee before lifting weights. Caffeine is a drug, albeit a naturally occurring one. It has definite fat-to-muscle benefit. Research indicates that not only does caffeine give an energy boost, it also helps muscles contract harder, because it stimulates the central nervous system and it helps burn more fat during exercise.

Caffeine actually induces the body to burn fat as an energy source during lighter exercise, sparing glycogen for higher intensity work. Tea contains more polyphenols than coffee, which are excellent antioxidants.

There are many marketers

Caffeine Content

Substance	Milligrams of caffeine
Coffee	
drip, 8 oz.	150-180
perked, 8 oz.	125
instant, 8 oz.	30-120
decaffeinated, 8 oz.	2-8
Tea	
Brewed, 8 oz.	20-200
Instant, 8 oz.	30-70
Soft drinks	
Mountain dew, 12 oz.	54
Colas, 12 oz.	36-46

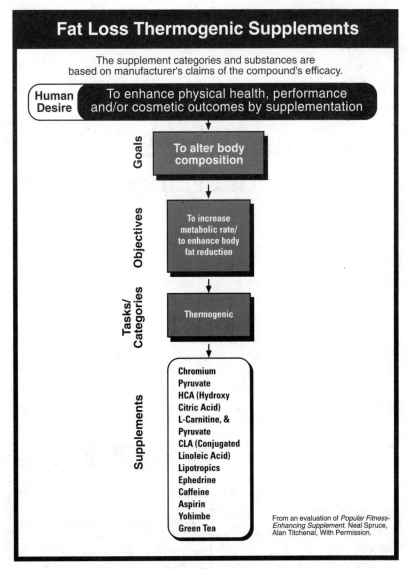

Fat Loss Thermogenic Supplements

The supplement categories and substances are based on manufacturer's claims of the compound's efficacy.

Human Desire — To enhance physical health, performance and/or cosmetic outcomes by supplementation

Goals — To alter body composition

Objectives — To increase metabolic rate/ to enhance body fat reduction

Tasks/ Categories — Thermogenic

Supplements —
Chromium
Pyruvate
HCA (Hydroxy Citric Acid)
L-Carnitine, &
Pyruvate
CLA (Conjugated Linoleic Acid)
Lipotropics
Ephedrine
Caffeine
Aspirin
Yohimbe
Green Tea

From an evaluation of *Popular Fitness-Enhancing Supplement*. Neal Spruce, Alan Titchenal, With Permission.

providing "mega-doses" of stimulants who would have us believe they have discovered the secret to miraculous body fat loss. There are several compounds that accelerate metabolism and body fat loss, but by far, the most effective is ephedrine.

Ephedrine is the active ingredient in an extract that comes from the herb ephedra, also called MaHuang. Ephedra has been used in China for at least 2000 years—primarily to treat ailments such as typhoid fever, arthritic pains, coughing, swelling of the ankles, asthma and even colds and flu symptoms. In fact, many of today's over-the-counter decongestants and cold medications contain ephedrine, the active ingredient in ephedra. It is the most common weight control product on the market today. Ephedrine speeds up the metabolism, raises body core temperature and accelerates calorie expenditure, all of which, over time, enhance fat loss. Marketers have refined the plant to its most powerful constituents, creating a powerful, brutish stimulant.

These stimulants are especially dangerous for those with high blood pressure, heart disease, thyroid disease or diabetes. When used with any other stimulants, over-the-counter or prescription drugs or certain supplements, they may be lethal. It comes as no surprise that Metabolife, one of the largest companies marketing ephedra, is now under criminal investigation for allegedly failing to disclose known dangerous side affects of the product to the FDA.

These "hopped up" stimulants are at best a "temporary" fix, like dieting. You may lose weight at first, but soon the products lose their "kick". Many users need to take more and more until they stop working entirely. Whipping our adrenal glands and central nervous system into overdrive often results in adrenal exhaustion (also known as burn out), which can put you into a metabolic prison from which there is no escape. The results are rapid weight gain and loss of energy, which is just the opposite of what you want to achieve!

Other popular thermogenic (heat-producing or fat-burning) products include Metabolife, Hydroxycut, Metabolean, Animal Cuts, Diet Fuel, Metabolift, Ripped Fuel and Hydrocut. Regardless of what name these stimulants are marketed under, check the label to see if they include ephedra or MaHuang.

Green Tea

There are two elements in green tea extract that act synergistically to stimulate thermogenesis – an antioxidant flavonoid called catecin, and caffeine. Green tea extract does not increase heart rate or raise blood pressure, so it is safe to use with most cardiovascular conditions.

When there are effective, safe, natural thermogenic supplements available, such as carnitine, Yohimbe and green tea, why roll the dice with potentially dangerous supplements?

	STIMULANTS Examples: ephedra and kola nut standardized extracts	ENERGIZING NUTRIENTS Examples: carnitine CoQ10, lipoic acid, green tea Yohimbe
Method Of Energy Increase	Stimulate central nervous system	Natural: promote optimal function of energy pathways in the body
Addictive	Yes	No
Quality of Energy	Jittery, stimulant energy	Natural, even energy
Short-Term Effects	Initial energy burst, then fatigue	Natural increase in energy that only improves over time
Long-Term Effects	Burns out adrenal glands; long-term use lowers energy and possibly immunity; may accelerate aging process	Increase energy with no adverse effects. Increase immune function; may slow aging process
Other uses	Ephedra can offer acute relief from asthma attack	Optimize many aspects of mitochondrial function; promote heart health; quench free radicals; maximize cellular health
Side Effects	Worsen hypertension and diabetes; promote and/or aggravate arrhythmias	None
Normal Constituents of Human Metabolism?	No	Yes

How hopped up stimulants can put your body into adrenal exhaustion.

❓ Fiction
Ephedra based thermogenics are safe and excellent for reducing body fat.

❗ Fact
Ephedra based thermogenics are dangerous and a "temporary" fix at best for losing body fat.

chapter 46

Juggling Your Hormones

A study of the functions of hormones could fill a library. Hormones monitor mineral and fluid levels and control digestion, metabolism, sexuality, moods and many other vital bodily functions.

Hormone replacement therapy (HRT) for Estrogen, Testosterone and Human Growth Hormone (HGH) are all options available from your doctor – but don't mistake any kind of HRT for an easy medical solution for getting fit. People want to believe they can just buy fitness in the form of a pill or shot. You can't buy fitness at the supermarket, the stock exchange or the doctors office – you have to work for it.

HRT, as it relates to fitness, should be used only if you have a medical problem that can't be fixed with diet and exercise, and only as a last resort. Juggling your hormones is an extremely delicate seesaw that can easily be thrown out of sync.

Estrogen

Even common HRT for menopausal women, using the hormones estrogen and progesterone, was recently proven to have unhealthy side effects. Federal health researchers say they have developed strong evidence that often hormone replacement therapy for healthy menopausal women does more harm than good, increasing a woman's risk of breast cancer, heart disease and stroke. According to Ross Prentice, a principal investigator on the study with Seattle's Fred Hutchinson Cancer Research Center, "It's disappointing we didn't find any (heart)-protective effects." This goes against years of conventional medical thinking that such drugs improve heart health.

If you are considering, or are currently on HRT, talk to your doctor to be certain that it is right for you.

Testosterone

As we age, most of us lack the energy we used to have. For men, the problem is often "low testosterone syndrome" (LTS). Men gain fat and lose muscle, may lose sex drive and motivation and often become depressed. Several factors can contribute to LTS, including alcohol, emotional stress, physical inactivity, smoking and obesity. Excess body fat, especially in the midsection, is the most common factor in LTS.

Testosterone is essential for many basic functions of the body. It is necessary to maintain high energy levels, bone mass and libido, and for increasing muscle mass and lowering body fat. It also contributes to improved concentration and memory – and even stimulates hair growth.

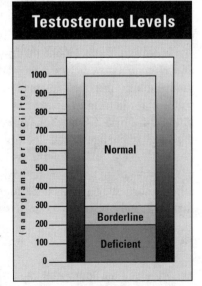

LTS is thought to be a contributing factor to Alzheimer's, a devastating disorder that strikes many older adults. Scientists have recently discovered that testosterone supplements in older men and women suffering from LTS help prevent the chemical deposits of chemicals called beta-amyloid peptides in vulnerable parts of the brain. These deposits are thought to be a primary cause of Alzheimer's disease.

As we age, our testosterone levels may be only slightly lower than when we were younger, but our biologically available testosterone is considerably lower. This means the testosterone is still there, but it doesn't work as well as it used to.

Have your testosterone levels checked with a total serum testosterone test. If it's low, weight training, a healthy diet and supplements will usually increase it to normal levels. If that doesn't work, seek your doctor's advice.

Over four million men in the U.S. whose bodies don't produce enough testosterone now take a doctor-prescribed synthetic version, mostly by self-injection, every one to three weeks. The synthetic version cannot begin to mimic the body's own management of testosterone levels. Side effects include a roller coaster of physical and emotional effects, including anger, depression and increased libido in the first few days, followed by lethargy and depression.

The latest, and easiest, doctor-prescribed method is an easy-to-apply testosterone ointment, AndroGel. Applied once or twice a day, the results are a more even plateau of testosterone, avoiding the ups and downs. Testosterone replacement therapy is still relatively new and has been known to cause the growth of prostate tumors or enlargement of the prostate. This is why men with low testosterone should consider replacement therapy only as a last resort.

"Andro" & DHEA

Other popular precursors for raising testosterone levels include androstenedione or "andro" (which Mark McGuire made popular) and Dehydropiandrosterone, known as DHEA.

Testosterone and DHEA levels peak in the late 20's to early 30's and decrease thereafter. There is ongoing research regarding these precursors abilities in people over the age of 40 to increase physical and psychological well being. Although there is no doubt they raise testosterone levels, there hasn't been enough research to determine how safe they are.

Like steroids, most precursors to elevating testosterone levels are banned from most sports organizations including the International Olympic Committee, the National Collegiate Athletic Association, the National Football Association and Natural Bodybuilding Associations. Unlike steroids, these precursors are both legal and available over-the-counter as of this writing, but this may soon change.

Human Growth Hormone – The Fountain Of Youth?

Human Growth Hormone (HGH) is touted by some to be the new fountain of youth and by others to be highly risky. According to Paul

Jellinger, the president of the American Association of Clinical Endocrinologists, "It is an interesting hormone, and we're learning about it, but the full effects of it as we age are far from known."

Stanley Slater, deputy director of geriatrics at the National Institute of Aging agrees, saying, "This is exciting as a research area, but there continues to be no proven clinical utility as an anti-aging compound."

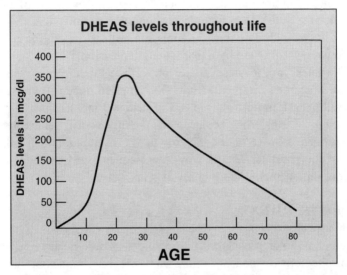

Here's what we do know: HGH is produced by the pituitary gland and, like the name implies, it is responsible for growth. The body's natural HGH levels start to peak during adolescence, when accelerated growth occurs. After age 30, the output of HGH declines about 14% per decade, so that total daily growth hormone production is reduced dramatically with age.

In numerical values, people produce about 500 micrograms of growth hormone daily at age 20, 200 micrograms at age 40 and 25 micrograms at age 80. At age 50, growth hormone production is only about 35% of that produced at age 20. Obesity, disease and surgery can also contribute to HGH deficiencies.

Doctors first began prescribing HGH about 35 years ago for children who were in need of a growth boost. It was first extracted from cow carcasses, but several incidents of children contracting mad-cow disease prompted synthetic production in 1985.

It's expensive and is now an "in thing" for the wealthy (no one else can afford it). The program usually begins with a comprehensive evaluation of nutritional, metabolic, immune and hormonal tests. These tests are followed by hearing and vision screenings, bone-density scans, treadmill stress tests and mind/brain assessments.

The testing reveals deficiencies in any number of areas, such as a thyroid condition, a blood sugar imbalance or osteoporosis. The costs for these tests range from $1500-$5000. Monthly fees for the supplement, which is injected, can cost upwards of $1000-$1500 a month and isn't covered by health insurance. Considered potent only when injected (as opposed to pills or sprays offered over the internet or in magazines), HGH advocates promise many benefits.

These same advocates are getting rich promoting their promises of lower blood pressure, increased muscle growth without exercise, increased skin elasticity, thicker hair that won't gray, sharper vision, restful sleep and increased sexual potency. The top seller of HGH, Genotropin, had sales of $461 million last year.

There is absolutely no scientific evidence to support any of these claims. There is evidence, however, of potential side effects from injecting something into the body that makes everything grow, including the heart and internal organs.

HGH may also stimulate tumor growth and tumors are more common as we age. Other side effects may include joint pain, carpal tunnel syndrome, fluid retention, insulin resistance and other cancers. Because we are trying to increase our muscle-to-fat ratio, HGH may sound very tempting, but there's much more to consider than muscle synthesis alone.

Medical research has revealed that the aging pituitary somatotroph cells can still secrete as much growth hormone as the young somatotroph cells if they are adequately stimulated. This has led some researchers to theorize that the reason for the decreases in HGH secretion must lie in the factors that regulate its release.

Weight training stimulates the pituitary gland, the thyroid and the entire central nervous system, providing increased levels of natural HGH, testosterone and endorphins.

Fiction
Human growth hormones slow the natural aging process.

Fact
There is no scientific evidence that human growth hormones have any beneficial effects to slow the natural aging process.

chapter 47

Step 6: Lifestyle

Being fit doesn't mean we're healthy. Health is based on three things – body, mind and spirit. Simple choices we make each day – how we handle stress, how we eat, if we drink or smoke, if we exercise, how well our family and social relationships affect us – all have major influences on our health and longevity.

A 300-pound overfat obnoxious jerk can dramatically change his physique, but he will still be an obnoxious jerk (albeit, a buff jerk). Without spirituality, we are incapable of achieving the incredible love and joy that life offers us. This is sort of like building a luxury ocean liner without a rudder or a high performance sports car without spark plugs.

Stress is a leading cause of poor physical and mental health. When we are under stress, our bodies release the stress hormone, cortisol. This hormone causes the proinflammatory immune factor IL-6 to be excreted. IL-6 exacerbates auto-immune disorders and other inflammatory conditions, and immune deficiency diseases. For instance, the HIV virus uses IL-6 to replicate itself. This powerful inflammatory immune factor also pulls calcium from the bones into the blood, causing osteoporosis.

Women are more prone to stress than men. With families, jobs, housekeeping and a never-ending list of miscellaneous tasks, they are often damaging their immune systems without even realizing it.

Women are also shallow breathers, which results in poor oxidation of the blood, increased stress levels and decreased immunity. Take several deep breaths in through the nose and out through the mouth many times per day to relieve stress and tension. This is a common practice for those who practice yoga.

The following serenity prayer, which is said at every AA meeting, is my favorite and a good way to deal with life.

The Serenity Prayer
"God, grant me the serenity to accept the things I cannot change, the courage to change the things I can and the wisdom to know the difference."

You can change and improve your body, mind and spirit. The mental aspects of training and self-improvement are by far the most significant. Don't expect others to make you happy. Happiness comes from within. Have confidence in yourself to achieve your goals. Physical, mental and spiritual well being will be your constant companions.

Suppliers Directory

- Ab bench 1-800-341-0103
- www. agelesstraining.com
- Apex Fitness Group, 1-805-449-1330
- Beverly International, 1-800-781-3475
- Bill Pearl Ent., www.billpearl.com or e-mail bill@billpearl.com
- Body View Advanced Diagnostic Scanning, Clackamas, Oregon 503-653-7226
- Body Gourmet Spice Blends 310-661-7761, or wwwflavorbank.com
- Bowflex, www. Bowflex.com
- Botox, Dr. Bruce Chisholm, Palm Desert, California, 760-779-9559
- Clarence Bass' Ripped Enterprises, fax. 505-266-9123, e-mail: cncbass@aol.com
- Health Scan Imaging, Palm Desert California, 760-674-8800,
  e-mai: info@healthscanimaging.com
- Jack and Elaine LaLanne, www.jack lalanne.com/biograph.html
- Lifelong Fitness, Bob Delmonteque, 1-800-323-4772
- Men's Fitness, 800-521-0303
- Master Trainer, e-mail: ageless.athletes@pcr-inc.com
- Muscle Media Magazine, 303-384-0080, www.musclemedia.com
- Muscular Development, 800-835-2246 ext. 500
- Natural Bodybuilding, 212-947-4322
- Naturally Ripped News, www.rippednews.com
- Natural Muscle Magazine, www.naturalmuscle.net
- Nature's Best, Isopure Protein, 1-800-345-BEST, Northwest 360-606-6996
- Personal training, www.bodlyfitnessbyjoyce.com, new.isagenix.com,
  e-mail: 2joyce@mail.com, p.o. box 4411, Palm Desert, Ca. 92261
- Personal training, Train with Frank Zane, 1-800-323-7537, www.FrankZane.com
- Personal Training Certification, Dr. Bob Delmonteque,
  International Sports Sciences Assn. 1-800-892-4772
- SayersBrook Bison Ranch, 1-888-472-9377, or www.sayersbrook.com
- The Fitness Revolution, books & supplements, 1-877-581-8276,
  www.thefitnessrevolution.com
- Thorlos Socks, 1-800-438-0286, or e-mail: srobideaux@thorlo.com
- Powerblocks, 1-800-446-5215 or www.powerblock.com

Glossary

Aerobic exercise. Prolonged, moderate-intensity exercise that requires less oxygen than your cardio-respiratory system can replenish to the working muscles. Burns body fat for energy needs.

Amino acids. Organic compounds that generally contain an amino and a carboxyl group. Twenty alpha-amino acids are the subunits which are polymerised to form proteins.

Anaerobic exercise. Exercise that uses up oxygen faster than the body can replenish it to the working muscles. Uses glycogen (muscle sugar) for energy needs.

Bodybuilding. Weight training applied with proper nutrition to alter physique.

Burn. A beneficial burning sensation experienced when training, caused by toxin buildup in the muscles.

Carbs. Carbohydrates

Cheating. Using less than perfect form when performing weightlifting routines.

Circuit training. A weight training routine that incorporates numerous exercises with a minimum of rest between sets. Increases aerobic conditioning, muscle mass and strength.

Cut. Refers to a bodybuilder with a high degree of muscle definition due to low body fat

Cutting. Refers to the process of reducing body fat by dieting.

Density. A combination of muscle mass and muscle density with low intermuscular fat.

Flexibility. A full movement of muscle tissue, connective tissue and joints that permit total suppleness.

Forced Reps. Upon failure of a movement, your training spotter takes a small amount of weight off to allow a few more repetitions of the movement.

Free-Weights. Barbells, dumbbells and related weight training equipment.

Growth hormone. Polypeptide (191 amino acids) produced by the anterior pituitary that stimulates the liver to produce somatomedians 1&2.

Growth hormone-releasing hormone (GHRH). Hormone produced in the hypothalamus that promotes production of human growth hormone.

Hormone. A naturally occurring substance secreted by specialized cells that affects the metabolism or behavior of other cells possessing functional receptors for the hormone. Hormones may be hydrohilic, like insulin, in which case the receptors are on the cell surface, or lipopholic, like steroids, where the receptor can be intracellular.

Human growth hormone. (Somatotropin). A protein produced in the pituitary gland that stimulates the liver to produce somatomedins, which stimulate growth of bone and muscle.

Lifting Belt. A leather or nylon belt 4-6" wide at the back that adds stability to your midsection when doing heavy lifts.

Metabolism. All the chemical reactions that occur in your body, all the reactions that take place in your brain, liver, digestive tract, muscles, heart, lungs and every other tissue or organ.

Muscle Failure. A point where muscles are fatigued and cannot complete another repetition of a movement.

Nutrition. Eating healthily to promote greater health, fitness and muscular gains.

Peptide. A compound of two or more amino acids where the alpha carboxyl group of one is bound to the alpha amino group of another.

Personal Trainer. A trained fitness professional who works with you during your weight training routine. Advises you on type of exercises, how to perform them, routines to follow, diet and supplements.

Pituitary. An endocrine gland located at the base of the brain, in a small recess of bone – certain sections of the pituitary secrete important hormones, including growth hormone and anti-diuretic hormone.

Precursor. Something that precedes.

Pump. When muscles become engorged with blood after intense training.

Repetition or rep. Each individual count of an exercise that is performed. Series of reps are called sets.

Resistance. The actual amount of weight you use on any exercise.

Rest Interval. The brief duration between sets allowing your body to partially recuperate.

Routine. Also referred to as schedule or program.

Safety Clamps. Clamps that secure a weight to a lifting bar.

Set. A group of repetitions followed by a rest interval.

Spotters. People who stand by to act as safety helpers when performing exercises.

Spot. Assisting those performing lifts.

Supersets. Alternating two exercises with no rest between sets and a normal rest between supersets.

Supplements. Concentrated vitamins, minerals, proteins and other nutrients to improve quality of diets.

Symmetry. The shape of a person's overall body appearance.

Total Failure. A point where you cannot move the weight at all; beyond failure, which is when you are unable to perform another full repetition.

Warm-up. Aerobic activity and stretching before weight training, often used to "warm-up" muscles.

Weight training. A general term used to define exercise utilizing all forms of resistance training.

Wheel. Weights of different sizes that slide on a lifting bar.

References

1. Chandra, RK. Fed Prae. 1 980; 39: 3088
2. Stamler J. et al. J Amer Assoc., 1986; 256: 2823-2828
3. *Best of Health* Stop Aging, pg. 200 Dr. Colgan
4. *All Natural, Muscular Dev*. Stop Aging 202, 3-98 Best of Health, Dr. Colgan
5. G. Erikssen, et al. "Changes in Physical Fitness and Changes in Mortality." Lancet 352 (1998) 759-762
6. A Gulide to Low Cholesterol Living, Human Health Division 1990, Drames Communications
7. J.R. Stout, et al. "The effects of a supplement designed to augment creatine uptake on exercise performance and fat-free mass in football players.", Med. Sci. Sports & Exerc. 29.5 (1997): S251
8. *Nutrition Almanac* by Lavon J. Dunne., USA FDA, T-Factor Diet by Martin Kethahn, Ph. D.
9. Bailey, Covert, *The New Fit or Fat*, Target Diet, Smart Exercise
10. Weider, Joe, *Ultimate Bodybuilding*, The Master Blaster's Principles Training and Nutrition
11. Applewhite , Roger, *Personal Trainer*
12. J. Anderson and B. Deskins, *The Nutrition Bible* (New York: William & Morrow & Co., 1995)
13. *Muscle Media 2000*, Bill Phillips
14. Will Brink, *Musclemag*, Measuring Body fat
15. Fat to Muscle, *Ironman*
16. *Cholesterol in Some Common Foods*, American Heart Assn. of Washington
17. JAMA October 4, 1955, Elevated Plasma Homocysteine Levels
18. The Colgan Institute, San Diego, California
19. Appleton, Nancy *Lick the Sugar Habit*, Penguin Putnam
20. Scientific American, Muscle, Genes and Athletic Performance, Sept., 2000
21. Gannett News Service, Get Your Body fat measured
22. Universal Matters, Ron Kosloff, Research Nutrition
23. Wolinsky, Ph.D. Professor of nutrition, Dept. of Human Resources, Houston, Texas
24. Universal Maters, Dr. Peter Fong, staff physician, Maxing it out, the Endomorph
25. Bass, Clarence, The Plains Truth, August Muscle & Fitness 2000
26. Ironman, The Creatine Edge, May, 2000
27. American Council on Exercise & American College of Sports Medicine, 1996
28. Oregonion, August, 2000, FDA & Food Labeling
29. The Atkin's Diet, Muscle Media, May, 2001
30. Better Nutrition, January, 1999
31. Muscle Media, July/August, October 2001
32. USA Weekend, How fat-free foods can make you fat, Feb., 2000
33. The Carnitine Miracle, 2000
34. Runn, Lola, The low-down on Liquid
35. Trainers' Desk Reference, Apex Fitness Group, 1st edition, 2000
36. Master Trainer-Ageless Athlete, March, 2001
37. The testosterone effect, Time, April, 2000
38. Alternative Medicine, March 2002
39. Miller, Colagiuri, Wolever, Foster-Powell-*The Glucose Revolution*
40. Apex- Trainers Desk Reference
41. Appleton, Nance *Lick the Sugar Habit Counter*
42. The Carnitine Miracle
43. Mature Outlook, August 2000
44. Storm, Mason-The Value of Vitamins, Max Muscle
45. Turner, Lisa-Power of the Plate-the 10 top antioxidant foods
46. Met-Rx Owners Manual, 1999
47. Health & Nutrition, The Low Down on Liquid, Runn, Lisa
48. Better Nutrition, Supplements Guide, 1999
49. Dr. Peter Fong, Universal Matters, 1999
50. Healthy Immunity, Stress: at the root of women's health issues
51. Social Gerontology: Biology of Aging-2001
52. Scientific American, 2000, Muscle-Genes and athletic performance
53. Robbins, John, *The Diet Revolution*
54. Universal Matters, Breathing and Heart Rate Control, Dr. Ton Seabourne, Fall 2000
55. Keep Pumping Iron, Aging doesn't have to result in loss of bulk, Elena Volpi, M.D., Ph.D.,
56. Food and Drug Administration "Final Rule" for Sucralose, 21 CFR Part 172, Docket No. 87F-0086
57. Labare MP, Alexander M. Microbial cometabolism of sucralose, a chlorinated disaccharide, in envirnmental samples. 1994 Oct; 42; 173-8.
58. Hunter BT. Sucralose. Consumer's Research Magazine, Oct. 90, Vol. 73, Issue 10, p57
59. Optimal Wellness Center, Dr. Joseph Mercola, Dec. 3, 2000
60. The Oregonian, July 9, 2002, Andy Dworkin
61. What if it's all been a big fat lie? Gary Taubes, The New York TImes
62. Nourishing Traditions, Sally Fallon with Mary G. Enig, Ph. D.

A Word From The Author

Jerry Hogevoll

As I neared my 50th birthday, a lot of bad things were happening in my life. I had worked hard all my life to build a good family life, a good business and become financially independent. Then everything took a turn for the worse. I got divorced, I was in trouble with the IRS, my Dad became very ill, my business was failing and my cholesterol was very high. My life was a roller coaster of stress, mood swings, anger, depression and unhappiness.

I put my faith in God and made the decision to get in the best shape of my life, not only physically, but spiritually as well. I made major changes in my diet, quit drinking and started lifting weights. Within six weeks I saw impressive results and 90 days later I had gone from 21% to 9% body fat. Not only had I transformed my physique, I increased my mental and spiritual well being. The stress in my life was still there but I dealt with it much better. My cholesterol dropped from 277 to 162 and I threw my cholesterol medication away.

My friends couldn't believe I made such dramatic changes in such a short period of time. Today, five years later, thousands of people across the country have dramatically improved their lives on the *Muscle & Longevity* program. Helping people help themselves is my reward. Every day I get calls, e-mails and letters from people across the country thanking me for helping them. I hope this book inspires you to make the decision to get fit and join *The Fitness Revolution.*

May God grant you health, fitness and happiness.